Quality
Smart Consumers

Strategies to save your money, time, and health

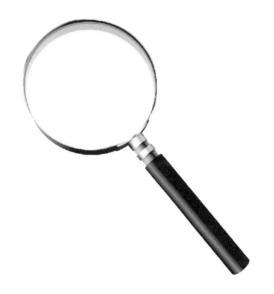

Rita A. Rooney, BSN, MPH

Healthcare-Equalizer.com

Rita Rooney
cell 571-723-5131

A Note to the Reader:

CONTENTS

Acknowledgements   1

Introduction   3

Part I: The Present Healthcare System

Chapter 1: A Broken System   13

Chapter 2: Transparency and Accountability Can Work   36

Part II: Take Charge of Your Health

Chapter 3: The Health Triangle and Your RNA Plan   53

Chapter 4: Prevention Core: Managing Your Health Risks   108

Part III: Take Charge of Healthcare Decisions

Chapter 5: Quality Healthcare Information   133

Chapter 6: Transparent Healthcare Navigation   168

Chapter 7: Your Healthcare Rights   210

Part IV: Take Charge of Monitoring Price, Quality, and Safety

Chapter 8: Price: The Elusive Factor in Healthcare 226

Chapter 9: Consumer Monitoring and Reporting   254

Part V: The Future

Chapter 10: The Best is Yet to Come   272

Healthcare-Equalizer Consumer Bill of Rights   292

ACKNOWLEDGEMENTS

This book is dedicated to my parents who taught me and my six siblings the importance of intellectual curiosity, hard work, human dignity, honesty, always doing your best, and giving back to your community.

My Dad had a framed quote in his 1950s "home office" – his basement sanctuary from life with an Irish Catholic wife and seven kids!

There's a better way. Find it. Thomas A. Edison

My Mom always stressed the golden rule in life and our universal rights for human dignity and compassion. When I recounted my work stories about advising patients with important health decisions, she often remarked to me, "Rita, how can you help the others that don't contact you? Well, Mom, this book is my best effort to help others!!

My gratitude extends to my husband, Frank, who inspired me to develop a Healthcare-Equalizer Consumer Bill of Rights for this book. This will be presented in Chapter 7. My husband, an experienced IRS tax attorney, introduced me to the IRS Taxpayer Bill of Rights. This taxpayer protection was the result of Congressional hearings in 1998 to investigate complaints of abusive behavior by IRS employees. Today, that Taxpayer Bill of Rights has been updated in 2014 and it is always included in any correspondence you receive with the agency.

Thanks so much to our three adult children, my siblings and extended family, friends, and professional coworkers for their support and encouragement. A special thanks to my good friend and fellow nurse, Nanette Hotchner, for excellent editing and professional inspiration. I have always taught our children to dig your heels in for the principles and values that matter most to you – those are worth the good fight. This is my "good fight." Please join me.

INTRODUCTION

My Dad was a physicist. The scientific method was his problem solution method of choice. He taught us how to apply the scientific principles - research, testing, analysis, and evaluation – to our household decisions. Whether it was finding the best cleaning product or the safest and most reliable car, we always read *Consumer Reports* before we made our purchase!

My Dad invented unit pricing for us! I vividly remember crouching in the aisles of Safeway in the 1960s crunching paper and pencil numbers on the total price divided by the total ounces of desirable snack foods. Dad only approved it as a smart value to buy after checking my math calculations. Our home taste tests later determined which brands and food products were our best buys!

Later in high school, my biology teacher explained how the scientific method, a deductive decision process, led to scientific discoveries that helped mankind. In college, I was introduced to the Nursing Process which parallels the scientific method. Our nursing professors drilled the importance of carefully written **SOAP** notes in the medical records. Our **Subjective** observations, **Objective** biometric measurements led to our nursing **Assessment** and **Plan of care**. My Dad and I enjoyed lively debates about the evaluation process built into this method on our 2 hour drive back and forth to college each fall and spring. It delighted me that his revered scientific method had convinced me of the power of measurement and evaluation to make wise decisions and improve things in life!

My first professional job as a Clinical Nurse with the National Institutes of Health (NIH) in 1975 was both inspiring and challenging. I looked forward to joint medical and nursing rounds as the team discussed how best to care for our patients on three month clinical research trials. Our staffing levels were excellent and patient education was an expectation within our primary nursing care model. Each primary nurse created a written nursing care plan to guide the care of her/his patients when she/he was off duty. There was so much we wanted to teach our patients – the requirements of their clinical trial, how to live with a serious uncommon disease, how to safely take new drugs and treatments, and how to control their disease so they could enjoy a better quality of life. We included family members in our discharge planning sessions and sent our patients home with written instructions and hoped for the best. Fortunately, we never had to worry about the cost of the care since NIH was federally funded and "free" for patients!

As I rotated work assignments between the inpatient and outpatient clinics at NIH, I became curious about how our patients managed at home. Did they take their medications appropriately? Did they adopt the healthy habits we recommended? Did they monitor their symptoms and communicate these changes to their doctor quickly to prevent complications? Did our patient education efforts really improve the healthcare outcomes in our clinical trials? Were our patients enjoying a better quality of life?

When I met with our patients in their follow-up outpatient visits, I had an opportunity to assess how successful our patient education efforts had been. It became clear that patient education improved our patient's health outcomes and quality of life after participating in our clinical trials. My professional focus shifted to learn more about quality healthcare and how to achieve it. I wanted to learn how to improve what wasn't working. So, I decided to pursue graduate school.

Studying at Johns Hopkins University in 1979 was a transformational experience for me. The Master of Public Health rigorous 64 credit curriculum taught me the benefit of interdisciplinary teams, shared global perspectives, and a public health mandate to deliver quality care in a prevention-based delivery system. My understanding of the healthcare system was broadened with courses in Epidemiology, Health Economics, Community Health Planning, Aging in America, Legal Issues in Healthcare, and Operations Research.

Graduate school group projects helped us practice collaboration skills as we problem solved common public health problems. I began to appreciate the influence of cultural, religious, and personal values as we designed and measured effective and efficient patient education programs. Our studies proved that patients who actively took part in their plan of care goals had better care outcomes. We discovered how asthma and diabetic education programs prevented emergency room visits and improved the patient's quality of life. We learned about the public health mandate to promote quality of care using a prevention based model of care and evidenced based guidelines to promote healthy communities.

Following graduation, I joined Georgetown University Hospital as the Manager of a federally funded Breast Cancer Patient Education Project. The focus groups with newly diagnosed breast cancer patients taught me how critical it is for patients to have accurate, current, and easy to understand disease and treatment information so they can make informed choices. The nine patient brochures developed under this grant were augmented with a train-the-trainer professional program on breast self-exam for doctors and nurses. My personal reward was empowering these women with information that gave them confidence in their ability to make informed decisions about life-altering surgery and other treatments. Despite a life threatening diagnosis, I could empower them to become a cancer survivor instead of a cancer victim.

My next professional challenge was to design and develop public and professional education programs. I chose to work with two non-profit foundations, The Asthma and Allergy Foundation of America (AAFA) and later, the National Osteoporosis Foundation (NOF). Listening to patient concerns as they faced serious chronic diseases enlightened me. I soon began to understand how chronic disease scared patients and threatened their quality of life. They wanted to manage the disease better and avoid costly complications and hospitalizations and enjoy life.

Designing patient educational materials taught me several things:

Understanding and treating the root cause gives the best control

A proactive approach to chronic disease improves quality of life

Action plans serve as blueprints for self-care management

It was a privilege to coordinate the First Asthma Patient Conference promoting self-management of chronic asthma using peak flow meters, medications, and environmental control methods. Self-management of chronic diseases was very effective once patients had the right information and an action plan to follow. They could take charge of their chronic disease once they understood the risks it posed to their health and quality of life. Then, they were eager to treat the root cause, measure and evaluate early symptoms, and stop flares sooner. Information was powerful and patient education meant better quality of life.

During my years with AAFA, an Asthma Action Plan was developed. This written collaborative plan between the patient and a healthcare provider taught them a biofeedback system to make smart decisions and self-manage their disease. Asthma patients like me understand that asthma flares have triggers. Our job is to identify the known triggers like include indoor and outdoor allergies, exercise, chemical odors, and environmental factors like smog. However, asthma also has silent triggers like bacteria and viruses. The classic symptoms of coughing, wheezing, and chest tightness can be dramatically reduced once we understand the root cause, control our triggers, and respond to early lung changes.

The AAFA Asthma Action Plan framed the concept of self-management around the stoplight color system. This easily recognized and popular theme introduced a method for asthmatic sufferers to take charge of their disease and be in the driver's seat! The Action Plan is actually a written blueprint for future decisions and actions. Once adopted by our patients, we were able to demonstrate decreased emergency room admissions and lost days from school or work.

What I have learned as a mild asthmatic has helped me get excellent control of a serious lung disease. I want to share this action plan approach to other chronic disease patients and motivate them to achieve better control of their condition. Self-management of chronic diseases is rewarding and successful. In chapter 4, we will explore this further.

My current professional nursing position with Medstar, Georgetown University Hospital in Healthcare Referral has given me an opportunity to interact with patients and providers across the Washington DC metropolitan area as well as across the country. Our office facilitates emergency transfer admissions as well as counsels patients about second opinion visits and other important healthcare decisions. Our daily transfer admissions remind us what the caboose of healthcare can teach us. Uncontrolled and untreated chronic diseases can cause hospitalizations and preventable deaths. End-of-life care discussions and decisions need to be front and center in families and in hospitals every day. Clearly, the healthcare engine needs to change and lead us forward to a prevention based system which stresses quality of health and life. Better health outcomes can be achieved at lower cost with more transparency and accountability to the consumer.

The Institute of Medicine 2011 Report on "The Future of Nursing" recognized nursing as one of the most versatile occupations in health care. Nurses have the scientific knowledge about diagnosis and treatment, but they also have roles to assess and triage acute needs, plan care, monitor care, coaching skills, teach patients self-care skills, support caregivers, and coordinate medical, community, and social resources. Their traditional holistic perspective makes them a key player to advance patient engagement trends in healthcare. Nurses attend to patient comfort, preferences, psychosocial needs, and the interplay between family and communities.

Recent studies document the success of nurse led collaborative teams to deliver quality patient outcomes, reduce emergency room admissions, and decrease hospitalizations in patients with multiple chronic diseases, and conditions.

High patient satisfaction scores are the high stakes reward in modern healthcare administration. This is where nurses excel due to their assessment, coordination, and patient education skills. As an academic liaison with the Catholic University School of Nursing in 2002, I gained an appreciation for the important role that graduate trained advanced practice nurses play in our healthcare system. Nurse practitioners deliver direct care services to consumers in a variety of care settings and earn high customer satisfaction scores and excellent care outcomes. Nurse educators train staff nurses and promote nursing research to evaluate the best nursing standards of practice. With our present healthcare reform efforts, nurses become key players.

The public trusts nurses! The December 2013 Gallup poll has again confirmed that NURSES are the most trusted profession with the highest ethical standards in the US! Nurses earn the public's trust daily. A new documentary on the American nurse is aptly titled, "From the first breath to the last,…" Today, nurses manage care across the lifecycle and advocate for healthcare consumers and healthcare quality and safety. Finding a "smart nurse" is often given as solution to patients having trouble discussing concerns with the medical staff.

Finally, my Irish Catholic roots and Jesuit influence have instilled a strong conscience to do the right thing and earn my professional integrity by delivering quality, transparent, and accountable healthcare services for all consumers. A beloved Bioethics pioneer, Dr. Joseph Pelligrino, recently passed away at age 92. The Georgetown University Center for Advanced Study of Ethics was recently renamed in his honor. One of his memorable quotes is, "Medicine is a moral enterprise, and if you take away the ethical and moral dimensions, you end up with technique. The reason it is a profession is that it is dedicated to something other than its own self interests."

Chapter 1: A Broken System

It may seem a strange principle to enumerate as the very first requirement in a hospital that it should do the sick no harm.

Hospitals are only an intermediate stage of civilization, never intended to take in the whole sick population. May we hope that the day will come… when every poor sick person will have the opportunity of a share in the district sick nurse at home.

…The Nursing of Hospitals must be done to …. satisfaction … And we may depend upon it that the highly trained intelligent Nurse …. Will do this better than the ignorant …."

Florence Nightingale

Do you hear the people sing?
Singing a song of angry men?
It is the music of a people
Who will not be slaves again!

"Do You hear the People Sing" *Les Miserables*

Our 21st century American healthcare system is broken. We have unacceptable levels of medical errors, medication mistakes, high costs, confusing and deceptive insurance plans, and excessive fraud without the best quality care outcomes. Fixing it is urgently needed. It is my opinion that the healthcare system and marketplace lack transparency and accountability to the consumer. Quality healthcare is about safe, desired care that is affordable, and accessible. It is also about a long-term smart economic investment of our healthcare dollars that values effective and efficient delivery of needed services. Many forces have converged on the US healthcare system and marketplace and led it astray from these goals. Let's find out what ails our present healthcare system of delivery as well as the business marketplace that supports it.

As a professional registered nurse with over 40 years of experience, I can attest to a broken healthcare system that no longer serves the consumer well. You are probably well acquainted with its inefficiency and lack of coordination: long waits to get an appointment, numerous voicemail options to leave messages at your doctor's office, confusing coded hospital bills and explanation of benefit (EOB) reports, long turnaround times to receive medical records, test results, and prescription refills. Unexplained surprise charges on your bill like facility fees and billing errors cause confusion and financial worry. Then, there are the more dangerous problems like medical errors and other safety concerns like preventable deaths.

There are serious larger issues plaguing the American health care system that we will explore in this chapter. My trademarked name, Healthcare-Equalizer, was designed to demonstrate to the public that there are things you can do and say to make our health care system accountable to us and improve our quality of care. Together, we can reform our healthcare system and build a consumer driven one. This book demonstrates how healthcare transparency, illustrated by the magnifier, can lay the foundation for accountable and quality care today.

Now, let's explore what's wrong with our present healthcare system.

Commonwealth Fund Report

This enlightening report takes a critical look at the present American health care delivery system and market and how we fare globally. The Commonwealth Fund is a private foundation that aims to promote a high performance health care system with improvements in access, quality, and efficiency. This mandate is served by supporting independent research on health care issues and providing grants to improve health care practice and policy. The Fund also has an international program in health policy to stimulate innovative practices and policies both in the US and globally. This 2014 global health care survey examined 11 high-income industrialized countries including Australia, Canada, England, France, Germany, Netherlands, New Zealand, Norway, Sweden, Switzerland, and the US. This survey of 20,045 adults focused on their experiences accessing and affording health care in their respective nation. The authors recommend their findings be viewed as a baseline to compare the performance of the US health care system against other nation's health care systems as the US system undergoes tremendous changes.

Here are some of their significant findings:

US ranks **lowest in infant mortality** and **highest for expenses**

For the **past 10 years**, the **US health care system** has been the **'outlier' – more costly, less accessible, less affordable** – and disturbingly, **lacking better health care outcomes** despite our excessive costs.

37% of US adults **went without recommended care, didn't seek care when sick or failed to purchase prescriptions due to the cost of that care.**

23% of US adults had **serious problems paying medical bills or were unable to pay them,**

41% of US adults spent **$1000 or more out of pocket for care in the past year, the highest in the world.**

32% of US adults spent time dealing with **insurance paperwork, disputed or denied claims, and questioned lower payments by insurers.**

75% of US adults said the health care system **needs fundamental changes or needs to be rebuilt.**

US has the **highest per capita rate, $8508**, compared to the next two highest spending nations, $5,669 in Norway and $5,643 in Switzerland.

US has the **highest insurance administrative cost, $606 per person.** This **110% higher administrative costs** is a symptom of our **complex and fragmented health insurance system.**

US and Canadian **adults reported longer waits for primary care and higher use of hospital emergency rooms**.

27% of US adults reported **no dental care in the past two years** and **33% reported going without dental care due to the cost.**

Who Killed American Healthcare?

Regina Herzlinger is a Harvard DBA economist and author of the 2006 book, **Who Killed American Healthcare.** She believes transparency is one of the key success factors in the US economy. Knowing the prices and quality of the goods and services we buy allows us to become "smart shoppers" in most every industry except healthcare. The real issue is economic power. The less you and I know about the cost, the **greater the economic power of those who do know.** In healthcare, those in the know include hospitals, insurers, pharmaceutical companies, and medical device makers. Dr. Herzlinger warned that such marketplace dynamics are hazardous to both our health and our nation's wealth.

The Bitter Pill: Why Medical Bills are Killing Us

Steve Brill's March 4, 2013 Time cover story, "The Bitter Pill," revealed the powerful influence of money in our healthcare system. Mr. Brill, an attorney and journalist founder of Court TV and now, CEO of Journalism Online, conducted a seven-month investigation of hospital billing charges using the well-respected healthcare research team of McKinsey and Company.

The surprising report findings include:

$2.8 trillion US healthcare market is a seller's market with unknowing consumers that can't negotiate what they don't know

US hospitals have a **secret internal pricing system,** the **charge-master,** a huge computer file.

25% of our **excessive healthcare spending** is **overpayment for services!** This represents **20%** of our **GNP,** twice as much as other developed nations

Hospital/provider billing error rate is as high as 80%

$5.36 billion spent in healthcare lobbying since 1998 is 3 times the defense lobbying efforts (Center for Responsive Politics)

69% of medical bankruptcies were for insured members.

62% of all bankruptcies are related to **illness or medical debt**.

US drug prices are **50% higher than other countries.** We spend $280 billion just on drugs.

This 7 month investigation following the money in American healthcare came to some stark and troubling conclusions:

The healthcare marketplace has transformed our 2900 tax-exempt "non-profit" hospitals into the community's most profitable businesses and largest employers and most highly compensated executives. They earn higher average operating profits than the 1000 for profit hospitals! Hospitals maintain this upward spiral by marketing efforts to attract new patients, raise prices, and increase bill collection efforts. With non-transparent prices and less competition, it can quickly dominate the local marketplace.

The secret hospital "chargemaster" system bears no objective rationale for its prices. Medicare reimburses for actual costs not the billed costs sent to patients. Private insurers broker discounts with less markdowns than Medicare. Uninsured self-pay patients are billed at the highest rate. Welcome to Healthcare Economics 101!

The most expensive healthcare marketplace in the world does not deliver better health outcomes for our expensive GDP investment. Yet, this healthcare mega empire (doctors, hospitals, nursing homes, health services, and HMOs, pharmaceuticals and medical device companies) like the profitable status quo! So, expect transparency and accountability changes to occur slowly. US healthcare providers order more very expensive CT tests than other nations. In fact, the use of CT scans in emergency rooms has quadrupled in recent decades.

Such technologic advances have made American care more expensive. Out healthcare system incentivizes such equipment because providers and manufacturers earn high profits and commissions.

Medical device implantable surgeries commonly bill 2.5 times the actual cost of the device and can sometimes generate a profit margin of 150%! Mr. Brill contends that the usual argument for more tests to prevent litigation is not necessary. Rather it is an excuse to increase profits since courts allow doctors a "safe-harbor" defense if they follow recommended practice guidelines.

In fact, a 2012 Government Accountability Office (GAO) report found the lack of transparency and extreme variation in hospital reported costs for implantable medical devices raises questions about whether they are achieving the best prices possible. An earlier 2008 Inspector General Report revealed that physicians routinely receive substantial compensation from medical device companies through stock options, royalty agreements, consulting agreements, research grants and fellowships. Within two weeks of the publication of this eye-opening investigative report, the former HHD Director, Kathleen Sebelius, released Medicaid and Medicare price and expense data.

Finally, Americans learned from the McKinsey research team that Medicare is actually putting the brakes on runaway hospital, provider, and drugs. Medicare is the only player in this healthcare market that has to balance its costs and answer to Congress and the taxpayers for wasting money. The other players, hospitals, drug companies, and insurers don't have to answer for trying to hold on to money it shouldn't. In a real market, all players usually have to balance countervailing interests.

Perverse Incentives

Dr. Marty Makary is the author of the 2013 book, **Unaccountable: What Hospitals Won't Tell You and How Transparency Can Revolutionize Health Care.** He left medical school because he didn't like the medical culture at the time because they didn't tell patients the truth. So, he enrolled in the Harvard School of Public Health, where he met researchers from around the world forming a new discipline in medicine – healthcare quality.

About a year later, he decided to re-enter medical school and become a cancer surgeon.

In his book, Dr. Makary examines the collateral damage of modern American healthcare – **uncoordinated care, poor quality, and low accountability to the consumer.** He coins the term "perverse incentives" to describe the profits generated in a system of care built on volume services using a fee-for-service model which he thinks incentivizes bad care.

Here are some of his conclusions:

Hospitals generate profit from complications sometimes as much as 10K

Our **medical industry rewards volume oriented services** instead of being accountable for performance like other industries

US doctors are **taught a subtle bias toward action and treatment** instead of watchful waiting and patience. The gray area of when to treat **incentivizes volume based expensive treatment options**

Both our **healthcare crisis** and our **2008 bank crisis** were **incubated** by an **unaccountable culture** of **rewarding short-term profits** using a lack of transparency and accountability. American medicine has fostered overtreatment and runaway healthcare costs and big hospital bills

These perverse incentives also include financial strings attached to research study results as well as unwanted care recommendations. We will explore more about this problem in future chapters.

Medical Mistakes

A 2010 *New England Journal of Medicine* study on medical mistakes concluded that 25% of all hospitalized patients will experience a medical error of some kind. That's one in every four patients or **100,000 patients harmed a year**!! Medical mistakes are not only far more common that they should be – they are a devastating cost burden on our health care system. Medical mistakes incur a tax on society by costs passed on in the form of higher medical bills, higher insurance premiums, and higher deductibles. The cost of these mistakes is also passed on to taxpayers (consumers) in the form of **rising Medicare costs**. A Forbes article in 2012 cites a cost of **$400 million.**

Corporate Public Relations (PR)

Insurance companies are not blameless either in this broken and poorly performing American healthcare system. **Deadly Spin** is a book written by Wendell Potter, an ex-insurance company insider with Humana and Cigna Insurers.

Potter believes corporate public relations (PR) is killing health care and deceiving Americans. As a senior public relations executive or "spinmeister" for 20 years, he admits his job was to enhance the reputation of the insurers.

Here are some of his revelations:

The **number one priority for insurance companies is enhancing shareholder value.**

The insurance industry **fattened our uninsured rolls by their past recission policies** which selectively **removed high cost insured members**

Private health **insurers abhor transparency and public accountability regarding claim denials, underwriting rules, payments to doctors and hospitals, death rates, racial or ethnic disparities** in health status or the **health outcomes of their members**. They protect this information as their trade secrets and label them "proprietary information".

The growth of **corporate power restricts choice for American healthcare consumers**

Opaque Prices

Recently, a recent Washington post article in December 2013 entitled, **"Hospitals can tell cost to park, but not of treatment"** cited the results of a *Journal of the American Medical Association* **(JAMA)** study on this lack of price transparency in healthcare. This study replicated a larger study using callers who represented uninsured customers.

They inquired about the costs of the following: an EKG, a hip replacement, and hospital parking.

Here are the results:

Only **parking fees** were **freely given** to the callers.

10% gave the **cost** of a **hip replacement procedure.**

15% gave costs for an **EKG.**

Such opaqueness in getting pre-treatment estimates makes it difficult for smart consumers to plan for expected healthcare expenses.

Most consumers make large purchases such as cars, appliances, home repairs, and remodeling projects with written estimates. Their wise decisions are usually based on what they need or want and can afford. Healthcare decisions should be made in the same manner.

Unwanted Care

Another problem in the US health care system is
"unwanted care." This is care that you don't ask for, but is
suggested or ordered by your doctor or health care
provider. We all experience it, many times unknowingly.
The bottom line for the consumer is unwanted care is
profitable for providers.

My first encounter with unwanted care occurred during an
annual gynecology visit one summer to discuss sleeping
difficulties as I entered menopause. I offered my self-
treatment strategy of a small dose of evening benadryl to
improve my sleep and quell my seasonal allergies. My
gynecologist expressed concern that the Benadryl might
"be addictive" and asked me to consider an alternative, a
new estrogen patch, because it had the "added protection
against some temporary cognitive changes that some
women experience during menopause". Her
recommendation annoyed and surprised me given my
family history of estrogen positive breast cancer and my

expressed desire to remain hormone free during menopause. I quickly reminded her of this despite the fact she had treated me for the past 10 years. Maybe her cognition was impaired I thought, but certainly not mine!! I asserted my desire to find a hormone free solution to my sleep problems. She continued making notes in my chart and left the room.

A few minutes later, the nurse returned and asked if she could apply the estrogen patch to my arm as she handed me the written prescription. I politely refused the prescription and dropped the opened patch in the trashcan. I told the nurse to let my gynecologist know I would not be returning next year. My beloved primary care provider was able to do my annual well woman exams and agreed to never prescribe hormones. A recent check on the website, www.probulica.org, revealed my gynecologist's annual financial string (about 80K) from the estrogen dot manufacturer!

My second encounter with unwanted care occurred with my allergy physician. After an ER admission for an asthma flare, I consulted a pulmonologist to get better control of my frequent sinus infections which seemed to fuel my asthma. The pulmonologist diagnosed mild asthma and recommended a full allergy workup.

Both indoor and outdoor allergies were the culprit or "root cause" of my sinus infections and asthma flares. So, allergy immunotherapy (allergy shots) for 5 years was ordered. After starting weekly shots, I initially saw marked reduction in my nasal discharge and stuffiness, less headaches, and less need for asthma medications. I graduated from the weekly shots to the monthly regimen. During my annual visit in year 3 of the 5 year plan, my allergist suggested some newer medications to take in addition to my solo prescription, a nasal steroid spray. I queried him about why he recommended new medications which I had not requested.

My allergist was annoyed by my comments stating "You ask too many questions. Besides, "I take these drugs and they can improve your breathing." I pointed out that my clinical exam and breathing results were great and I was enjoying a high quality of life with daily exercise without asthma symptoms, less work days lost to sinus infections, and more restful sleep patterns. My impression was the allergy shots were just what I needed to keep my asthma and allergies well controlled. My allergist kept writing while I discussed my refusal with him and just handed me the two prescriptions as I exited the office.

I dropped the prescriptions in the trashcan and he followed me out of the exam room and apologized for the delay in the serum being ready. I was asked to see the nurse practitioner for my remaining two annual visits. She remarked, with a smile, what a great response I had to the allergy shots. She asked whether I had any annoying symptoms to discuss. I commented that my allergic eye symptoms were still a problem and she tweaked the serum vials to achieve better control. She also suggested wearing a dust mask while cleaning to reduce the nasal and eye irritation. This was very helpful. I completed my 5 year immunotherapy plan and now have excellent control of my asthma and allergies.

After visiting the www.propublica.org website, I discovered my allergist was handsomely rewarded by the two pharmaceutical manufacturers of the drugs he recommended for me! So it confirmed that "perverse incentives" created unwanted care recommendations which I refused. We will explore this concept of unwanted care in later chapters since it weaves itself into our care in silent and confusing ways. End-of-life care is another area of unwanted care that delivers expensive high tech care that doesn't improve health outcomes for many sick and dying patients. You will learn more about other options such as palliative and hospice care in Chapter 6.

Consumer Dissatisfaction

Now, let's examine the consumer perspective. A Harris Gallop poll in July 2012 revealed interesting results on experiences and opinions of healthcare consumers.

47% reported being **very satisfied** with their last office visit

36% reported being **somewhat satisfied** with their last office visit

29% satisfaction score with recent **health insurer** interaction

17% dissatisfaction with **healthcare provider visits**

Harris notes that these numbers contrast with other industries where high consumer satisfaction scores are usually given. For instance, 63% highly satisfied with their last restaurant visit, 62% with their online shopping purchase, and 59% with their last bank visit.

Harris also noted that it sharply contrasts with the **29% satisfaction score** for their most recent **health insurance** company interaction! The insurers have company with the low 28% mobile phone store visit satisfaction scores. The

17% dissatisfaction score (with **most recent healthcare provider visit)** was comparable to the same level of dissatisfaction with their mobile phone store visit at 18%. Personally, I can't help, but wonder if a lot of this dissatisfaction with insurers is about the lack of price transparency and accountability to the consumer as they make changes to their plans!! It didn't matter what kind of plan - phone, health or internet service provider – the **same business practice of elusive prices and unexpected changes in the plan drives the dissatisfaction.**

The Gallop poll asked consumers to rank the importance of factors driving a positive experience with their doctor and/or other healthcare provider.

83% rated the top issue as the **doctor's overall knowledge training and expertise.**

62% rated the **doctor's ability to access their medical history**

29% valued minimizing paperwork

My personal experience with unwanted care from my gynecologist attests to the importance of doctor's assessing a patient's medical history and care preferences. **In the end, consumers desire clinical training and expertise,** accurate, personalized health data, and face to face time with healthcare providers.

A November, 2014 Gallup Poll shed light on the fact that cost is still a barrier between Americans and medical care. This year **33% patients and families put off care due to cost. This is the highest level recorded by Gallop in 14 years** of reports. What was more disturbing is the **delayed care was for serious conditions**. That makes sense to me because more Americans have health insurance coverage which guarantees preventive care. Unfortunately, with more high-deductible plans and higher co-pays, more patients and families are unable to get needed care due to unaffordable out-of-pocket costs.

Here is the delayed care rate according to type of insurance:

57% for the uninsured

34% for private insured

22% for Medicare/Medicaid insured

Now, look at my Wall of Shame healthcare statistics

Adverse drug effects (medication errors) rate is about **1.5 million annually** with a **cost of $8,760**

100,000 medical errors and **180,000** Medicare patient deaths per year at **4.4 billion in 2009**

The **US** is ranked **37th (last place)** in the world on **health outcomes** and **50th on infant mortality rate**

$750 billion overspent annually on healthcare by the US compared to other developed nations

62% of personal bankruptcies are related to medical bills and **69% of** these are insured (IRS)

33% American families put off healthcare due to cost (Gallop Poll, 2014)

$280 billion spent 2013 on **prescription drugs** in US is double other countries cost

DHHS inspector general report for 2012 shows **1.2 billion recovered** in CSM fraud investigations

80% **error rate for hospital/ provider bills per** Medical **Billing Advocates of America**

128% **increase employee cost health premiums vs 38% wage rise and 28% rise in inflation**

So, let's summarize what ails our poorly performing American healthcare system:

Our disease oriented fee-for-service model of care incentivizes volume care, bad care, and unwanted care as well as skews some research study results

Our expensive healthcare system does not deliver "high value" care for consumers or "high economic value" for our nation

Consumers are dissatisfied with hidden costs, unsafe care, unwanted care, poor coordination of care, billing errors, unfair billing practices, and deceptive insurance plans and provider business policies

Chapter 2:   Transparency and Accountability Can Work

An educated consumer is our best customer

Sy Syms

I have an almost complete disregard of precedent and a faith in the possibility of something better. It irritates me to be told how things have always been done. I defy the tyranny of precedent. I go for anything new that might improve the past.

Clara Barton

It is true that peace treaties are sometimes signed by businessmen.

Antoine de Saint Exupery, **The Little Prince**

Sy Syms was a pioneer in the garment business who created a string of discount clothing stores in the 1980s. I enjoyed shopping there because he had a unique and transparent pricing system. Each clothing tag listed the price of the garment by date. The price decreased the longer it remained in the store. So, the customer could decide when to make their purchase. His motoo, "an educated consumer is our best customer," stressed what customers always want – transparent prices!

Unfortunately, the healthcare marketplace and its business practices have taken the opposite stance – offering consumers elusive prices, unacceptable medical error rates, narrowed insurance networks, higher deductible and out of pocket costs, healthcare fraud, and high billing error rates. These cause harm to consumers' physical and financial health and is unacceptable. It also results in unaccountable healthcare. We want quality, safe care that has high health and economic value for our hard earned dollars. So what is a healthcare consumer to do?

While writing this book, I was inspired by the "Les Miserables" musical and movie about the French Revolution. The lyrics from the "Song of Angry Men" echoed in my mind as I saw the American healthcare consumer fighting against bad care due to perverse incentives that valued volume driven profits over safe and evidenced based quality care. I thought, maybe we need a healthcare consumer revolution to reform and transform our poorly performing healthcare system!

The "Les Miserable" lyrics remind us that "there are things a people can do to overcome their power." Let's examine what those things are for health care consumers. My trademarked name, Healthcare-equalizer, emphasizes that there is an unequal playing field in the American healthcare system. Consumers must adopt a buyer beware attitude in the healthcare marketplace and understand their rights. Information is power and the current healthcare transparency movement is the consumer edge we need to take charge of our healthcare decisions and receive accountable, quality care.

First, let's learn what solutions have been proposed to reform our present broken healthcare system. The American healthcare system is a disease-oriented medical care system with a fee-for-service model that incentivizes volume care, unwanted care, and bad care. So, we need to reform our fee-for-service care model with a prevention based model which creates healthcare quality by rewarding healthy behaviors, treating root causes, and educating patients. Let's look at the evidence.

Solution #1: The Economic Argument for Prevention

The Milken Institute is a nonprofit, nonpartisan, and publicly supported group which issued a report in October 2007 on the state of America's health. Their research discovered that our gains in treatment outcomes for cancer and decreased mortality from cancer and heart disease are threatened by a dramatic growth in the percent of Americans diagnosed with diabetes and cardiovascular disease due to increased rates of obesity and inactivity. Unhealthy communities also drain our nation of worker productivity and strain our healthcare system with chronic diseases that could be prevented and diagnosed earlier.

The Milken Institute 2007 Report entitled "An Unhealthy America: The Economic Burden of Chronic Disease" charted a course to save lives as well as increase worker productivity and stimulate economic growth. Here are some of their research findings:

50% of Americans suffer from **at least one** of seven most common **chronic conditions** - cancer, diabetes, hypertension (high blood pressure), stroke, heart disease, lung conditions and mental health disorders. Each of **these chronic conditions** is linked to **behavioral and/or environmental risk factors** that prevention measures can address.

The Milken Institute predicts a possible **42% increase** in these seven **chronic diseases** for a   **total cost of 230.7 million plus $4.2 trillion in treatment costs and lost economic productivity by 2023.**

The **economic impact** on the US economy from **these chronic diseases** has been a staggering **$1.3 trillion annually!!** (1.1 million for lost productivity and $277 billion for treatment).

Cancer and hypertension pose the largest threat due to their prevalence rates.

The Milken Institute recommends a national commitment to a "healthy body weight" campaign to match our effective smoking cessation programs, and prevention initiatives to reduce alcohol consumption and improve physical activity.

The power of prevention is huge. **The Milken Institute projects the US can prevent 40 million new chronic disease cases by monitoring biometrics and public education programs about obesity and sedentary**

lifestyles. We can increase our **GNP by $905 billion due to gains in worker productivity,** and earn treatment cost savings of **$218 billion** annually! This translates to economic savings of 1.1 million reducing our GNP expenses by 27%!

The Milken Institute guidelines for change include:

Incentives in the health care delivery system to promote prevention and early intervention.

Employers, insurers, governments, and communities must collaborate and develop **strong incentives for patients and providers to prevent and treat chronic disease effectively.**

Increase health care spending for health promotion. This is consistent with the evidence of the effectiveness and efficiency of healthy lifestyles to reduce long-term healthcare costs.

This requires a national long-term commitment to a prevention based healthcare system and supports informed, educated consumers, healthy communities, and employers who take charge of their responsibilities to promote healthy lifestyles and behaviors.

Solution #2: The Affordable Care Act (ACA) and Accountable Care

The ACA has demonstrated an equalizer role in removing perverse incentives within our healthcare system by certain provisions in the law. Specifically, the healthcare protections mandated include: an umbrella over ten million more Americans who didn't have health care, prohibit exclusions for pre-existing conditions, eliminate co-pays for prevention care like immunizations, and end the annual lifetime caps by insurers..

This historic law also established a **Patient-Centered Outcomes Research Institute (PCORI)** to expand comparative-effectiveness research efforts. These efforts employ evidence from research studies to set effectiveness and efficiency rates for various drugs, diagnostic tests, and screening measures and then assign grades to the available evidence. Access to such objective and evidenced-based diagnostic and treatment information is badly needed by consumers and providers so informed and wise healthcare decisions can be made. Also, information that is independently evaluated by groups without financial strings can remove the financial "perverse incentives."

The ACA has changed the landscape of American healthcare. Integrated teams will care for patients and be held accountable for quality healthcare outcomes. They will also risk not being paid by Medicare for unnecessary re-hospitalizations. The hospital's quest for marketplace dominance will be abandoned because consumers will flock to the hospital with the best quality metrics for the care they desire. These changes are powerful consumer incentives. Let's take a closer look at the history of the ACA law.

In **2007** a landmark report from the **Institute of Healthcare Improvement** identified several problems. The **Commonwealth Fund**, a private foundation with a goal of promoting an effective high quality healthcare system, launched a **Triple Aim initiative: improve the health of Americans; enhance the patient/consumer care experience stressing quality, access, and reliability; and lastly, control and decrease the cost of care**. ACA is based on the results of these efforts to design a highly performing healthcare system that is prevention based, improves the health of Americans, decreases cost, and improves efficiency.

The Commonwealth report studied certain care organizations that they termed, "high performance delivery systems" or Accountable Care Organization (ACO). The ACO case studies found their success by promoting information continuity, patient engagement, care coordination, healthcare teams, continuous innovation, and convenient access to care.

The ACO concept was incorporated into this 2010 healthcare law. Since 2012, healthcare organizations can apply to the federal government to become ACOs for Medicare enrollees. The Centers for Medicare and Medicaid define ACOs as groups of physicians, hospitals, and other healthcare providers who come together voluntarily to offer coordinated high-quality care to their Medicare patients. **Coordinated care benefits patients by ensuring they get the right care at the right time, avoid medical errors, and avoid duplication of services**. The new healthcare law gives financial incentives to become an ACO. When the ACO provides high quality care and spends its healthcare dollars wisely, the ACO will share in the savings it generates for Medicare. These incentive payments will reward care expenditures below a specified benchmark amount as well as certain quality indicators.

Advocates of ACOs praise this system of care delivery to move the American healthcare system from a focus on **payment incentives for disease or illness to a focus on health and wellness**. This translates for the consumer as a **move from fee-for-service to a fee-for-value based care model to improve our healthcare outcomes.** As we discussed earlier, our fragmented fee-for-service model gives "perverse incentives" to volume based care which oftentimes leads to bad care outcomes, unwanted care, and runaway healthcare costs. Most likely, you have witnessed ACOs forming in your community. Hospitals and healthcare systems lead the effort and merge inpatient and outpatient care facilities into a coordinated network of physicians and providers. Future effectiveness and efficiency studies will evaluate whether they improve our health outcomes and also control cost.

ACOs will emphasize **care requirements** instead of **clinical diagnosis** used in a medical model of care. ACOs will create **care delivery units** focused on coordinated care across a continuum of care transition points. These transition points include **wellness and maintenance, minor illness, major acute illness, chronic intermittent care, and end-of-life care.** The effectiveness of the ACO design will be measured by optimizing health outcomes and efficient use of resources. Obviously, the ACOs will operate with highly committed multidisciplinary teams of care providers.

Here is a glossary of some new terms:

Medical Home or Patient Centered Health Home – These will replace the traditional primary care office with an integrated team of healthcare providers to include physicians, advanced practice nurses, care coordinators, social workers, nutritionists, clinical nurse educators, home health aides, nutritionists, physical therapists, community health workers and information technologists.

Care Coordinators – Most likely these will be nurses who will lead a comprehensive team of health providers who deliver care to a certain group of patients during their episode of care. They will seek to achieve desired health outcomes by standardizing care pathways as the patient transitions between different care settings.

Patient Navigators – Nurses may also take the lead in this area as well. The emphasis will be a proactive approach to managing a patient's trajectory toward better health outcomes across all levels including community visits and guiding patients through episodes of care.

Collective Accountability – This represents the new culture of accountability in our healthcare system. This emphasizes problem solving at all levels, forging a cooperative and collaborative relationship between clinicians and healthcare executives, and a quest for data, information, knowledge, and evidence.

Bundled care payments fortunately will replace confusing, complicated hospital bills in the future. ACOs earn a profit for delivering bundled price **"value care"** that delivers quality, safe, healthcare outcomes.

The Affordable Care Act gives Americans the right to purchase health insurance with tax-free income; creates public data about the performance of the healthcare system like price, safety, and quality; and gives the poor funds to shop for health insurance like everyone else. This law leaves the shopping decision for healthcare to the consumer. So, we need to be prepared for these new responsibilities and assume our vigilant role to keep a checks-and-balance in an often abused delivery system.

Solution #3: Transparency

Dr. Makary recommends price and performance data disclosure as a public good in which the government sets the standards. Herzlinger comments about the failure of voluntary disclosure among professional groups. She cautions that independent measurement by outside impartial parties is necessary to create honest and reliable performance metrics for quality, safety, and consumer satisfaction scores. **Performance metrics protect the patient and the community.** Future chapters will discuss more about how to use these metrics.

Such transparency can make the practice of medicine more honest and accountable to consumers. When consumers develop price sensitivity, the healthcare system becomes more highly performing. In fact, the Swiss healthcare system mails insured members a copy of their bills for any healthcare service received. This consumer oversight is most likely one of the reasons this Number 2 ranked (Commonwealth Report 2014) country only spends 12% of GDP compared to the US 20%! The Swiss also rank highest for healthy lives along with the French and Swedes. The US ranks last!

Dr. Makary also recommends breaking the institutional culture that exists in some hospitals. Replacing perverse incentives that stress volume care and high profits with **teamwork based best practices usually delivers quality patient health outcomes**. Dr. Makary, now a Quality Assurance Officer with Johns Hopkins Hospital, remarks that consumers can learn to avoid hospitals that are poor performers with high infection rates, medical errors, and repeat admissions. Quality performance metrics for the consumer draws attention to poor performers and draws business away from them.

Transparency extends to financial disclosures for doctors and providers to remove perverse incentives from care recommendations to patients. We will discuss financial transparency in future chapters.

Solution #4: Stopping the Deadly Spin

Potter, now a senior fellow at the Center for Media and Democracy, has excellent recommendations on how to spot spin propaganda, an unethical public relations tactic. Ethical PR builds and maintains mutually beneficial relationships between an organization and the public. It is two-way communication. Spin public relations is one-way communication.

Step One: Be aware of anything that **sounds too good to be true.**

Consumers must take a skeptical stance with such advertising. If it sounds too good to be true, it probably is!

Step Two: Be aware of techniques that **reframe a public debate to shift focus away from their client,** the provider or institution such as a hospital or insurer. Then, they introduce misleading information to dilute or redirect the controversy. Lastly, they use **philanthropy to overshadow negative publicity or unethical behavior by their client. These techniques promote an attitude**

rather than a product – such as extolling the virtues of a corporation or its contributions to society. By staying positive instead of negative, there is an implicit message that the company is making your life better in some way. This makes you want to support the company even when it is lying to the public, dumping toxic waste, or willfully marketing a dangerous product or good.

Step Three: Recognize the sinister tactic in the use of the **"third party technique."**

The support for a cause or product is shown by a front group unknown to the public. They usually have a mission statement to defend consumer's rights, but you need to find out who **the funders are**. Visit www.sourcewatch.org and find out. Potter is now a senior fellow on healthcare at the Center for Media and Democracy.

Solution #5: Educated and Informed Healthcare Consumers are Smart Consumers

The Healthcare-Equalizer advocates a consumer driven market with customers who reward service providers who deliver safe, evidenced based quality care that is free of financial strings, affordable, and accessible in our neighborhood. The rest of this book is dedicated to educate the consumer on how to navigate our "buyer beware" health marketplace and demand transparency and accountable services that give us the quality healthcare we want and need.

Such smart and wise healthcare consumers will need to master new skills and habits to transform our healthcare system and keep it safe, honest, and delivering high quality care at an affordable price. There are three important responsibilities that consumers must assume in this reformed healthcare system based on prevention: take charge of your health, your healthcare decisions, and monitor the price, safety, and quality of our healthcare system.

Take Charge of Your Health

Chapters 3 will give you information on the health triangle and you will learn tools and strategies to adopt healthy habits. Chapter 4 will teach you how to assess your personal health risks and create an action plan with your provider to minimize and control them.

Take Charge of Your Healthcare Decisions

Chapter 5 will help you find quality sources for a variety of healthcare information that you need to make smart and wise decisions.. Chapter 6 will teach you how to navigate a powerful and complex healthcare system that is slowly changing. You will learn how to save money, personalize your care, and avoid unwanted care. Chapter 7 informs you about your healthcare rights and introduces my Healthcare-Equalizer Consumer Bill of Rights.

Take Charge of Monitoring Price, Safety and Quality in Healthcare

Chapter 8 will examine how to budget for expected costs, comparison shop for price and quality to get your best health value, and teach you to beware of financial strings that influence your care recommendations. Chapter 9 discusses the important checks-and-balance role that smart consumers must play in our healthcare system prone to fraud, poor care, dangerous care, and unwanted care.

Finally, Chapter 10 examines the public health mandate for our communities and nation as we adopt a prevention-based model of care and create a highly performing healthcare system that delivers high economic and health value. Yes, there is a better way to deliver healthcare in America! This good fight is a challenge we must accept. It can bring us future dividends for our loved ones' health and quality of life. Let's learn how to make our American healthcare system great!

Chapter 3: The Health Triangle and Your RNA Action Plan

When health is absent, wisdom cannot reveal itself, art cannot become manifest, strength cannot be exerted, wealth is useless, and reason is powerless.

Hemophilus, Ancient Greek physician

Not only to be well, but to use every power that we have to use

Florence Nightingale

Health is a state of complete physical, mental and social well-being and not merely the absence of disease or infirmity.

WHO – World Health Organization

Now I will tell you a secret. It is very simple. It is only with the heart that you can see rightly; what is essential is invisible to the eye.

Antoine de Saint Exupery, **The Little Prince**

Health, as you can see, is so much more than not being physically ill or not suffering from a chronic disease or condition. The Ancient Greek quote at the beginning of this chapter laid the foundation for how important one's health is to living a good life – one filled with vitality, energy, strength, friendship, and community – the things that are most important in life, but invisible to the eye as St Exupery reminds us. Dr. Atul Gawande, author of **Being Mortal,** discusses his journey as a physician as he watches his father die. He discovers what really matters most in life is the patient's definition of quality of life. End-of-life care like all other healthcare services must support our personalized quality of life definition.

So, as consumers, we need to understand what contributes to our health and also understand what lifestyles and daily habits undermine our health in subtle yet predictable ways. These lifestyle habits - how we live in our homes, workplaces, and communities - either promote our health or progressively destroy our health over time.

Health is really a set of habits that confer good health as evidenced by our biometric measurements, (blood pressure, pulse, and weight), our feeling of energy and vitality, and our ability to work, attend school or take care of our families without disability from chronic disease.

The Human Body: Basic Physiology

Physiologists study the structure and function of the human body. As the preface to my Basic Human Physiology college textbook by Arthur Guyton reads, "the human body is one of the most complex and yet most beautiful of all functional mechanisms." Dr. Guyton succeeded in his desire to "excite" this "student to a lifetime of physiologic thinking." He amazed us with facts such as "each individual cell in our body has all the genetic components of the entire human being and a variety of control systems for thousands of chemical reactions within each cell." In fact, the human body consists of 100 trillion cells! Wonder what he would think about our new discoveries in genome sequencing!

Professor Guyton viewed disease as an "unplanned physiological experiment." He described diabetes in 1971 as a "pervasive disruption to all the physiological functions in the human body not just regulation of blood glucose, carbohydrate metabolism or fat metabolism." How right he was!! He taught us that our cells and body systems are interdependent. A moderate level of cell dysfunction leads to sickness and chronic disease. Severe destruction leads to death.

Guyton defines homeostasis as the "maintenance of constant conditions in the body or internal environment " This balancing act includes the role of our lungs to give oxygen to our cells, our kidneys to regulate electrolyte concentrations, our intestines to digest and nourish our body, and our heart to circulate cell nutrients. The human body is actually a machine that needs daily attention to achieve maximum performance. When we adopt healthy habits and manage chronic health conditions, we give our body the daily attention it requires to perform well. Our reward is a healthy, vibrant life.

Professor Guyton remarks that the "human brain carries within it a computer with capabilities and functions that all the electronic computers of the world cannot at present achieve." Please bear in mind that this book was written and published in 1971!!! Our 21st century information explosion on brain structure and function is assisted by new imaging technologies and neuroscience research findings. A prominent neuroscience researcher, John Medina wrote a book called, **Brain Rules.** Let's ponder his 12 brain rules as we strive to reach our optimum health and wellness.

Exercise boosts brain power. We actually improve our thinking skills by moving. Our brains were built to walk about 12 miles a day! Twice a week aerobic exercise cuts dementia risk by 60%

We actually have 3 brains: The brain stem or "lizard brain" keeps us breathing, the animal or "cat" brain controls the 4 F's – fighting, feeding, fleeing, and reproducing and the third "human" brain is our cerebral cortex or brain surface with its deep electrical communication pathways with specialized centers for speech, vision, memory/learning, and symbolic reasoning.

Every brain is wired differently. Learning physically changes the brain and these changes are unique to the individual.

Human brains thrive on novelty and discovery. We don't pay attention to mundane things. The brain's attention can only focus on one thing at a time and wasn't built for multitasking! When we are emotionally aroused, we learn and remember better.

Humans must repeat to remember. Practice, practice, practice applies to the brain and learning! When we reproduce the environment when we first learned something, we increase the chance of remembering it.

Long-term memories can take years to get fixed in the brain. During sleep, we now know the brain integrates new knowledge with past memories and stores them together as one.

We have a universal biological drive for an afternoon nap. Sleep loss and deprivation damages attention, executive function, working memory, mood, quantitative skills, logical reasoning, and motor skills.

Stressed brains don't learn the same way. Stress hormones – adrenaline and cortisol - are built for a fight or flight response to an imminent danger. The stress reaction impacts a child's ability to learn as well as an employee's productivity. So reducing chronic stress is important.

The brain learns most effectively when all or several senses are stimulated. Scents can evoke powerful memories along with visual media, photographs, and voice recordings.

Vision trumps all the senses. We see with our brains not our eyes. This dominant sense uses half of the brain's resources. We learn and remember best through pictures rather than written or spoken words.

Male and female brains are different structurally and biochemically. Women react to acute stress with more emotional detail than men.

BlueZone Health Studies

Now let's look at health around the world. In 1990, Dan Buettner, the founder of **Bluezones,** researched **areas around the world where people have the best longevity**. He coined the name, BlueZones, because he circled these geographic locations with a blue pen to identify them on a global map. Today, BlueZone researchers study the lifestyle and environments of these longevity communities.

They have identified **5 BlueZones:**

California, Loma Linda

Costa Rica, Nicoya Peninsula

Greece, Ikaria

Italy, Sardinia

Japan, Okinawa

The most recently identified BlueZone community, Ikaria, Greece, eats a Mediterranean diet which includes fruits, vegetables, whole grains, beans, nuts, fats, and fish. The tiny 99-square mile island nearly 30 miles off the coast of Turkey has 10 times as many siblings over 90 as anywhere else in Europe. Also, their rates of cancer, cardiovascular disease, depression, and dementia are lower than the rest of Europe and the men outlive the women.

My husband and I recently vacationed in beautiful coastal Sardinia, Italy. I can understand why longevity is great here – an active, friendly community with fresh, healthy food, great air quality, safe neighborhoods, calming blue waters, and beautiful green-scape living!

Dan Buettner has also identified **nine principles** of a Blue Zone Lifestyle:

Move naturally and **keep moving** instead of sitting

Know your purpose each day

Kick back against **stress**

Eat less. He recommends you stop eating when you are 80% full.

Eat less meat. Most centenarians diets have beans as their staple food.

Drink in moderation.

Have faith. Attending faith based services four times a month is a marker of living longer.

The **power of love is huge**. Longevity is associated with commitment to family and aging parents.

Stay social in your daily life. Your social network should support your healthy habits.

Buettner calls these longevity pockets around the globe "thrive centers" because they help us understand the physical, social, and psychological areas of our lives that have the greatest influence on our well-being or health. Staying active, eating a nutritious diet, being spiritual, cultivating friendships and a communal living experience all enhance our health and wellness. The BlueZones remind us that it is our personal quality of life definition that should direct our healthcare decisions. For more information, please visit his website at www.bluezones.com

A new book, **Blue Mind,** by marine biologist and conservationist, Wallace J. Nichols, explores a fascinating concept. He maintains humans have a deep connection with the deep blue that is biological. He has proven this by brain imaging tests which reveal that when we are see or hear water, our brain is flooded with our feel good hormones, dopamine, serotonin, and oxytocin. Stress hormone levels like cortisol decrease. In fact, our bodies are 60% water and our brain is 70% water. Nichols notes that **our brains prefer the color blue. Water appears to relax us and increase our ability to focus.** So, water is good for our health and seems to be a stress reliever! It is interesting that **all five BlueZone areas have close proximity to bodies of water.** Also, human babies grow in their mother's uterus, which is actually a bag of waters giving the fetus both buoyancy and protection from injury.

Healthy Habits Research

Since our 1st and 2nd causes of death in the US are heart disease and cancer, it makes sense to examine what the professionals who care for these patients recommend for having a good and long life. The consensus opinions from American and British medical experts from their respective National Heart and Cancer Societies stress 5 vital healthy habits:

Healthy weight – body mass index (BMI) 18.5-24.5kg/m

Regular exercise goal of 150mins/wk at a moderate pace

Healthy balanced diet

No Smoking

Low alcohol intake

The American studies have consistently shown that people who adopt 4 or more of these healthy behaviors or habits have a much lower chance of developing coronary disease, a slower progression of existing cardiac markers, and decreased incidence of cardiac events like stroke and heart attacks. Similarly, people with at least 4 of these healthy habits also produce a significant decrease in all-cause mortality including cancer deaths. A long-term (35 year) British study with a huge sample size also found that participants with at least 4 of the habits had a 60% decline in cognitive disorders and a 70% reduction in diabetes, vascular disease, cancer and death. **We always believed that what was good for the heart is also good for the brain and now we have proof!**

Most health studies emphasize our healthy biometrics as indicators of healthy lifestyles. Our healthcare providers measure our pulse, weight, blood pressure, and glucose levels during our physical exams to evaluate our health and wellness. These healthy yardsticks are the direct result of healthy habits. So, what do you think are the most important health habits to adopt?

The Health Triangle

There is a famous Aristotle quote, "We are what we repeatedly do. Excellence, therefore, is not an act, but a habit," that sums up this important point in health. Our health and wellness is reflected in our daily habits. A recurring theme in the obesity prevention literature is the health triangle concept. The health triangle **represents the interdependent influence of nutrition, sleep, and exercise as the prime determinants of your health.** Each of these habits is equally important in maintaining good health.

It makes sense that monitoring just these 3 daily habits should keep or move our biometric measurements closer to a normal range and thereby decrease our risk of developing a chronic disease. So, frequently measuring our biometrics and adjusting our healthy habits will help us detect changes that threaten our health. Remember, measurement and evaluation can improve things. A healthy lifestyle delivers healthy dividends!

So, I have developed a practical solution to apply the principles of the health triangle theory. My tool is called the **Healthcare-Equalizer Daily RNA Action Plan.**

Healthcare Equalizer: Daily RNA Action Plan

The health triangle promotes three healthy habits: Rest/relaxation, Nutrition, and Activity/exercise to build your health and wellness. RNA is the building block of the cells of our body so it seems logical to use the acronym, RNA, as our blueprint for our healthy habits for life! The corollary is also true, without these three healthy habits, you will likely decrease your quality of life. Let's explore what it is known about each of these important health behaviors.

Part I: R is for Healthy Relaxation and Sleep

The human body and mind need rest and relaxation. We just learned that the human body is a machine that needs both rest and relaxation to function optimally and reduce the incidence of chronic conditions. Life is full of stress that affects our body and mind and we must adapt to keep our health in balance. Stress can be physical, psychological, or mental. The health quotes at the beginning of this chapter remind us that we must balance the demands of our internal and external environments each day.

When our bodies are under stress regardless of its cause – physical or psychological – our body goes into the fight or flight mode. This mode is mediated by the parasympathetic or autonomic nervous system. Most of us know the classic stress symptoms – that revved up feeling we get when we are scared, worried, or just angry and frustrated! Our hypothalamus, at the base of our brain, releases two stress-related hormones, adrenalin and cortisol. Adrenalin gives us the rapid heartbeat and increases our blood pressure while cortisol increases our blood sugar and hinders our immune system response. Chronic stress hinders the function of the immune system and increases the risk of many health problems.

We now know that chronic stress puts us at greater risk of developing metabolic syndrome. This is a combination of several conditions – diabetes, high blood pressure, high blood sugar level, obesity and abnormal cholesterol levels. All these symptoms also increase the risk for cardiovascular disease. Chronic stress interrupts our sleeping habits which causes changes in our leptin levels which can trigger weight gain. So, chronic stress fits Dr. Guyton's definition of a body dysfunction. This leads to changes in the body and brain which increase our risk for illness and chronic disease. Chronic stress also undermines learning in children and productivity in adults. So, it makes sense that we learn healthy habits to manage our stress.

Health studies continue to find stress as a contributing factor in most conditions like cancer, heart disease, diabetes, depression, hypertension, and obesity. The Herbert Benson Stress Management Institute at the University of Massachusetts hospital claims 60- 90% of patient visits to primary care doctors are stress related. The World Health Organization (WHO) estimates that stress costs US companies about $300 billion annually due to absenteeism, employee turnover, and low productivity.

Many people react to stress with emotional eating and overeat or increase their consumption of high calorie "comfort foods" which are usually high in fat, salt, and sugar. Those foods make us feel better, but it can lead to obesity and overweight. Obesity can then lead to diabetes, heart disease, cancer and depression. Others react to stress by using alcohol to relax or caffeine to stimulate them.

This yoyo effect just taxes our adrenal glands to produce more stress hormones all day long. Many stress management programs emphasize the need for participants to calm the mind and body with relaxation methods, eat healthy balanced meals, and have a more active than sedentary lifestyle.

It has become quite obvious that the brain works in concert with the body. So, calming our brains and changing our thinking has demonstrable health benefits. For instance, exercise increases the brain's production of the feel-good neurotransmitters or endorphins – dopamine and serotonin – which improve our mood and consequently lower the risk of depression. These endorphins also prevent heart disease, stroke, diabetes, and cancer.

Stress Management

Relaxation is a form of rest for the human body. Many studies demonstrate that we don't devote enough time daily to this important concept of resting the body and mind. **The Relaxation Response** by Dr. Herbert Benson was first published in 1975 and introduced a controversial subject for Western medicine, self-healing for patients. As a young cardiologist, Dr. Benson was frustrated by medically treating his hypertensive patients with lifelong medications only to find them battling irritating side effects. He decided to investigate the relationship between stress and high blood pressure. His studies revealed new ways to self-regulate blood pressure without using drugs. Transcendental practitioners (T.M) approached him to collaborate on their research. Dr. Benson coined the term "relaxation response" to describe the startling physiologic changes that TM practice elicited – namely a drop in heart rate, metabolic rate, and breathing rate.

Dr. Benson suggested that stress released hormones-adrenalin and noradrenaline- caused many Western medical problems. His relaxation response was effective for hypertension, headaches, cardiac rhythm irregularities, premenstrual syndrome, anxiety, and mild to moderate depression. He started the Mind/Body Medical Institute at Deaconess Hospital in 1988 as a model of self-care techniques. Dr. Benson believes that humans are born with this relaxation response or a physiologic state of quietude. This is an essential survival mechanism because it enables humans to heal and rejuvenate their body. The relaxation response counters the powerful effects of the fight or flight stress response.

Meditation and Yoga

Meditation and Yoga are two Eastern Medicine habits that calm the body and mind. Recent studies have proven their value in **relieving stress and inflammation in the body**. We have always known these mind-body practices can lower your pulse and blood pressure. But newer studies with better brain imaging techniques are revealing more benefits and how they work. Mindfulness techniques help people concentrate on the present moment. Brain imaging and genomic studies have recently examined the changes in the brain and human body. Meditation actually changes the brain structures over time and changes the body's stress level as evidenced by changes in pulse and blood pressure readings.

What is most amazing is that **these mind body techniques also appear to switch on and off some** genes linked to stress and immune function. This is powerful information. Other recent studies have demonstrated that one session of relaxation-response practice enhanced gene expression involved in energy metabolism and insulin secretion and reduced gene expression linked to inflammatory responses to stress. Even novice meditation students experienced the effect. So, meditation works to lower our stress related changes in the body. Some researchers also think telomerase length of our cells can be lengthened by regular meditation. Telomerase length has been called the "immortality enzyme" for our cells. So, perhaps meditation reduces cellular stress related aging.

Relaxation breathing methods calms the heart and mind and makes it difficult for people to stay stressed. By remaining in the present, the mind pushes away past and future worries. Deep breathing methods emphasize **4-7-8 breathing**.

Breathe in through the nose for 4 seconds
Hold your breath for 7 seconds
Breathe out slowly through your mouth 8 seconds

This Ancient Indian breathing method is best done with your tongue placed behind your front teeth. If you practice this daily 2 times a day, you will experience changes in your anxiety and stress levels and also enjoy healthy blood pressure and pulse rates. The key to mastering this technique is to do it in a regular manner daily. Over time you may find it helpful to do this to get back to sleep, to prepare for a stressful meeting, or to reduce your anxiety about a situation.

A certain amount of stress in life is actually helpful, but when we encounter toxic stress in our lives, we need tools to cope. Yoga and meditation are two powerful and effective remedies.

Music

Music can calm us or stimulate us. After reading about my response to Les Miserables "Song of Angry Men," you probably already realize I love listening to music. It is my go to stress reliever next to exercise. Today, brain researchers are studying how the brain responds to music. Here are some of the exciting findings:

Listening to music lowers patient's pre-surgery anxiety and also decreases their cortisol levels, a measure of anxiety level. Listening to music is also associated with higher levels of immunoglobulin A and increased white cell counts, the cells that fight both germs and bacteria.

Listening to music illuminates a part of the brain called the nucleus accumbens. This is where the brain rates music and registers our likes and dislikes. Another part of the brain, the superior temporal gyrus, forms strong templates of songs we have heard in the past. That is why someone who grew up listening to Motown tunes, like myself, enjoys those songs more than my children!

Brain imaging scans have revealed that brain regions for attention, planning, and memory are activated when we listen to music. Perhaps, music teachers have always been correct that learning music helps us learn other things.. When we listen to music, we process sounds, memorize lyrics, and remember the melody.

Hospitals have found success offering string musicians to calm patients and providers. Harpists are particularly helpful in assisting dying patients and their families. Sound is the last sense that dying patients lose. Guitar players have helped chemotherapy patients cope with common side effects like nausea and vomiting. Perhaps, the music distracts the brain from feeling sick.

Dance, Humor, and Pets

We now have an extra reason to dance besides strengthening our bones and exercising our body - relaxing our minds! Have you ever noticed how people feel at a wedding reception when they come off the dance floor – relieved, exhausted, and smiling! Dancing to your favorite tunes can lower your blood pressure. Music creates a sense of community and unifies us as we enjoy it together.

Robin Williams portrayed Dr. Hunter in the 1998 box office hit movie," Patch Adams." The film was based on a book by Adams and Maureen Mylander entitled **Gesundheit: Good Health is a Laughing Matter.** Adams found his purpose in life using humor to bond with patients and treat them with compassion. He brought attention to treating both the body and spirit of the patient. Today, we know humor releases calming neurotransmitters in the brain as well as relaxes our blood vessels.

Numerous health studies have documented the effect of our furry friends and pets have on our blood pressure and sleeping habits. As Buettner describes in his BlueZones studies, healthy communities and human longevity are based on caring connections. Taking care of pets in our homes and stray animals in our communities give us a purpose each day. When we share pets and protect animals from harm, we shape healthy communities. Pets also bring much joy and contentment to prisoners, wounded warriors, and hospitalized children and adults.

Rest and Relaxation – the Forgotten Healthy Habit

Recent studies have illuminated the importance of a good night of sleep:

Helps keep a healthy weight level

Stabilizes our emotions and moods

Prevents accidents and arguments

Improves immune function

Maximizes our memory and thinking performance

Researchers believe our brain cells shrink during sleep so the fluid can be flushed more efficiently. The brain has only a limited amount of energy. So, either we are awake and aware or we use the limited energy to clean house at night! Proteins associated with Alzheimers disease and other neurologic disorders are removed more efficiently at night. So, don't skimp on sleep quality and length!

A recent BBC article suggested that the brain actually works as we sleep connecting neurons in various parts of the brain with neurons in other regions of the brain. This nteresting study will lead to further research on neuron connectivity and how the presence or lack of this connectivity may contribute to Alzheimer's disease and other neurologic disorders. Lesson learned – get a consistent good night of sleep!

Visit this cool BBC site called the sleep profiler. www.sleepprofiler.com/uk which helps you calculate your ideal number of sleep hours given your personalized information.

Now let's find out what the current sleep recommendations are:

National Heart, Lung and Blood Institute (NHLBI):

Newborns	16-18 hours per day
Preschool Children	11-12 hours per day
School Aged (6-12)	At least 10 hours
Teens	9-10 hours
Adults	7-8 hours

The National Sleep Foundation has very similar sleep recommendations for each age category as well. They report that only about a third of high school students get at least 8 hours of sleep on an average school night. Some sleep hygiene tips to improve your sleep include:

Keep a regular schedule of bedtime and wakeup time each day

Avoid large meals, alcohol, nicotine and caffeine within 2 hours of bedtime

Keep your bedroom cool and remove distractions like TV, cell phone and computer screens.

The Center for Disease Control and Prevention (CDC) 2013 Health Bulletin declared that "Insufficient Sleep Is A Public Health Epidemic." This lack of quality sleep has been linked to motor vehicle accidents, industrial disasters, medical and other occupational errors not to mention the irritability and arguments that tend to occur in sleep deprived persons! The Institute of Medicine encouraged collaboration between the CDC and the National Center on Sleep Disorders Research to monitor the incidence and prevalence of unhealthy sleep behaviors. A large 2008 survey sponsored by the Behavioral Risk Factor Surveillance team (BRFSS) had disturbing trends. This large sample size study with 74,571 adult respondents from 12 states found:

35% consistently slept less than 7 hours a night

48% reported routine snoring (a symptom of sleep disorders)

38% reported falling asleep unintentionally during the day

5% reported nodding off while driving.

The National Department of Transportation estimates that drowsy driving is responsible for 1,550 traffic fatalities as well as 40,000 nonfatal injuries each year. So, be sure to get a good night sleep!

Part II: N is for Nutrition for your RNA Action Plan

Healthy nutrition is an essential component to maintain good health, prevent illness, and treat disease. Eating is fuel for our body to build healthy cells and maintain their important functions. Not eating well makes the human body machine function ineffectively. Many health problems are related to poor quality diets and nutritional imbalances. Poor nutrition coupled with sedentary lifestyles hastens the development of several chronic diseases Including heart disease, stroke, diabetes, and cancer. Experts have projected **that 66% of deaths in the US are due to diseases that are directly influenced by diet.**

Nutrition Primer

The latest United States Department of Agriculture (USDA) dietary recommendations include the following:

7 servings daily of fruits and vegetables

Eat more lean meats and plant proteins daily

Eat more unsaturated fats and limit saturated fats

Eat more whole grain and whole foods

Drink more water instead of sugary drinks

The healthy plate design recommends 25% or a quarter of your plate should contain fruit and vegetable foods. The easiest solution is to have one serving of a fruit and one or two servings of vegetables with each meal. Other countries often serve vegetables with breakfast such as tomatoes, carrots, olives, and potatoes.

NUTRITION GLOSSARY

Bad and Good Carbohydrates

In 2002 the National Academies of Medicine recommended that we focus on getting good carbohydrates and fiber in our diet. The best way to get fiber is to eat plant foods such as **fruits and vegetables – the good carbs**! A good carb is:

Full of fiber

Slowly absorbed by the body

Doesn't spike our blood sugar level

So, healthy whole grains also qualify as good carbs. These include **quinoa, buckwheat, brown rice, barley, oats, amaranth and whole wheat.**

The **bad carbs** include **white rice, bread, and pasta as well as pastry and sweets** which are processed and refined to strip away the healthy fiber.

The CDC recently added a link to their fruit and vegetable calculator for you. This tool calculates the number of calories you need based on your sex, age, and activity level and then determines your ideal fruit and vegetable intake.

It actually quantifies what you need to eat each day and then also gives you examples of how to get that quantity. My results recommend 1.5 cups of fruit a day and 2.5 cups of vegetables a day. The tool gives you visual examples of what constitutes a cup of various fruits and vegetables.

A cup of vegetables serving:

> 1 cup of raw or cooked vegetables
>
> 1 cup of vegetable juice
>
> 2 cups of raw, leafy greens.
>
> 1 medium potato, 2 large stalks of celery, 12 baby carrots, 1 large sweet potato, or 1 large ear of corn

A cup of fruit serving:

> 8 oz of fruit juice
>
> ½ cup dried fruit
>
> Small apple, large banana, medium grapefruit, large orange, 2 large or 3 medium plums, 8 large strawberries or 1 large bell pepper

½ cup servings of common fruits and vegetables include:

> 4oz applesauce

16 grapes

1 medium cantaloupe wedge

½ medium grapefruit

4 large strawberries

5 broccoli florets

Please visit the CDC website https://www.cdc.gov and use the search box to find the fruit and vegetable calculator. It is quick and informative!

Healthy Fats

Fats provide the most concentrated source of energy and are essential for certain body functions. However, consuming the proper amounts of healthy fats is critical for the proper function of the circulatory and nervous system and normal brain development. Children under age 2 require the highest percentage of fats in their meals. The body uses saturated fats to make cholesterol.

Omega 3 and 6 fatty acids are naturally occurring healthy polyunsaturated fats. These essential fatty acids are **not**

produced by the body, but needed for its healthy functioning. So we have to eat foods rich in these fatty acids. These essential fatty acids reduce cholesterol levels and lessen inflammation which contributes to heart disease and heart attacks. Some studies indicate they improve the control of certain chronic diseases like asthma, multiple sclerosis, psoriasis, some liver problems, and promote positive mental health. Healthy wild fish sources include **mackerel, salmon, bluefish and albacore tuna.** Other sources include **nuts, seeds, and avocados and olive and canola oils.** A handful of walnuts, almonds, brazil nuts or peanuts a day is good for your heart and body.

Saturated Fats are hard at room temperature like animal fats in lard and butter. High intake of saturated fats can increase your risk of developing coronary artery disease. Other sources of saturated fats include **milk, cream, eggs, red meat, chocolate,** and **solid shortenings. Coconut oil** is a **healthy saturated fat** and **butter** contains compounds that are **cancer protective.**

Trans Fats are commonly found in margarine and shortening. The labels on these products list hydrogenated or partially hydrogenated vegetable oils which contain trans-fats. Trans-fats are very unhealthy fats. These fats are chemically processed to transform liquid fat to a solid fat. They are formed when you overheat liquid oils or reuse oil. Trans-fats are often used to preserve the shelf life of many prepared foods as well as in fast foods like pizza, potato chips, and bakery goods. **Trans-fats significantly increase your risk of developing heart disease by elevating your bad cholesterol level (LDL) and decreasing your good cholesterol level (HDL).**

Fiber

Fiber is found in whole grains **cereals and flours, brown rice, bran, fresh and dried fruits, nuts, seeds, flaxseed, lentils, peas, beans and vegetables**. These foods can be great to **maintain weight and help you feel satiated**. About 10 grams of fiber is found in 1 cup of cooked dried beans, peas or lentils or one half cup of wheat or oat bran. Leaving the skin on organic produce can increase the fiber and nutrient content.

The **benefits** of **fiber** are multiple:

Increase your metabolic rate including GI motility

Eliminate carcinogens and toxins which decrease colon cancer risk

Encourages less overeating by feeling more full

Prevent absorption of some fats which decrease bad or LDL cholesterol levels

Stabilize your blood sugar

Protein

Protein is used to **build our cells, tissues, enzymes, hormones, and antibodies.** Proteins also help maintain that very important fluid balance in the body, assist liver regeneration, reduce ammonia levels and help transport fats and fat soluble vitamins. Proteins are created by linking chains of nine essential amino acids. It is our very DNA. Essential amino acids can't be made by the body so **we must consume them in our food.**

Protein sources include **animal** foods like **meat, fish, poultry, eggs, milk, yogurt and cheese.** Grass fed and wild animals like **bison, wild turkey and venison** are **less processed** and healthier sources. **Plant protein** sources include **soybeans, quinoa, seaweed, dried beans, peas, tofu, kefir** and **seitan** as well as **nuts and seeds.** Vegetable sources tend to lack some of the essential amino acids so eating a variety of both animal and plant protein sources give us a more balanced diet. Eating too much protein can be dangerous and lead to leaching calcium from your bones and stress the liver and its function in removing toxins from the body.

Whole Foods

Healthy whole foods contain the whole food product compared to processed foods. Whole wheat flour contains the entire wheat grain. In contrast, processed white flour has less fiber and nutrients due to its chemical and physical processing. Whole grain foods are nutrient rich with phytochemicals, fiber, vitamins and minerals. Phytochemicals are antioxidants that are chemo-preventative which means they protect the body from developing cancer. These complex compounds are found in plants. The chemicals in plant pigments that give the plant its characteristic color are among the most potent. So, the deeper colored fruits and vegetables have greater antioxidant and nutrient quality. Whole foods don't contain preservatives, chemicals, and toxins. Some examples of **whole foods are raw fruits and vegetables, various nuts and seeds, and whole grains like millet, quinoa,**

buckwheat, brown rice, barley, oats, amaranth and whole wheat.

SELECTED NUTRITION TOPICS

Eating to Promote Immune Health

Our immune system interacts directly with the whole body and is not confined to a vessel or organ. It represents the internal defense system. The immune system is comprised of the spleen, thymus, and lymphatic tissue which produce interferon. Other important players in our immune function include the white blood cells, the lining of the intestines, and bone marrow. Stress affects our immune health. Stress can be exposure to toxins, poor diet, illness, and lack of sleep.

The health of our immune system is influenced by our nutritional state. A low fat, primarily vegetarian diet **rich in whole grains** is usually recommended. Perhaps this is why we see greater longevity in the BlueZone areas where a Mediterranean diet flourishes. Their immune systems are operating at high performance levels. **Low sugar intake** and **moderate protein consumption** are also helpful. All aspects of immune function are impaired when protein intake is deficient. **High intake of sugar actually reduces the activity of white blood cells.**

Obesity also impairs our immune system. The lymphocytes or white blood cells have reduced bacteria fighting abilities. Evidently, **elevated cholesterol and triglycerides reduce the immune response to an attack of bacteria and other foreign invaders** in the body and **reduce** the **efficiency of the antibody response. Excess alcohol** also **diminishes the immune system** of the entire body.

Vitamins and some trace minerals promote a healthy immune system:

Folic acid deficiency, the most common vitamin deficiency, **decreases the production of our white blood cells.**

Vitamin B12 deficiency also **reduces our immune response and antibacterial resistance.**

Vitamin A activates the natural killer cell activity and the antibody response. It also protects the thymus gland and can stimulate its growth.

Vitamin C helps the body resist infections and has antiviral and antibacterial action.

Vitamin E protects the spleen and thymus and is a potent free radical destroyer. It also activates T cells which defend the body against invaders.

Selenium and zinc also benefit immune health with zinc especially important to the health of the thymus gland.

Brain Health: The Mind Diet

A nutritional epidemiologist, Martha Clare Morris, PhD, at Rush University Medical Center in Chicago developed this diet which is a hybrid between the DASH (Dietary Approaches to Stop Hypertension) diet and the Mediterranean diet. Both of these diets have scientific evidence supporting their cardiovascular benefits from large randomized controlled clinical trials. We have already learned that what is good for the heart is good for the brain so it makes sense to use a diet to treat cognitive problems that also prevents heart attacks, stroke and high blood pressure.   Dr. Morris thinks the MIND diet is easier to follow than either the Mediterranean or DASH diets.

Here is how it works. There are 15 dietary components comprised of 10 "brain healthy foods" and five unhealthy foods.

The brain healthy foods include: Green leafy vegetables, other vegetables, nuts, berries, whole grains, fish, poultry, olive oil, and wine.

The unhealthy foods include: cheese, pastry and sweets, fried or fast foods.

The Rush Memory and Aging Project studies 923 Chicago residents and looks for factors that protect cognitive health. The study started in 2004 and is ongoing. The 2013 results revealed that moderate adherence to the MIND diet decreased risk of developing Alzheimer's disease by 35%. Surprisingly, moderate adherence to the Mediterranean diet or Dash diet showed no reduced risk for Alzheimer's. However, participants who closely followed the Mediterranean diet had a 54% lower risk for Alzheimer's and close followers of the Dash diet had a 39% reduced risk for Alzheimer's. The study also found that the longer the participants followed the MIND diet, the more protection against Alzheimer's.

Food Preparation

The quantity and quality of fats in our daily meals is important to prevent many chronic diseases. Fats can increase or decrease inflammation in the body which leads to various illnesses and diseases. When foods are fried, the high temperature converts the healthy fats to unhealthy fats. Nutrients can be best preserved when foods are eaten raw, steamed or baked. Raw foods contain the highest amount of vitamins and nutrients. So bring on the celery and carrot stick snacks!!

Another factor in food preparation is limiting pesticide exposure on fresh fruits and vegetables. The Environmental Working Group, http://ewg.org publishes a "Dirty Dozen" list each year. It has named apples, strawberries and grapes the dirtiest and at the top of the clean list are avocados, sweet corn, and pineapple. Consider using a fruit and vegetable scrubbing brush and/or vegetable based washing rinses before eating fresh fruits and vegetables that you buy in supermarkets. Better yet, grow your own!

Herbs and Spices

Most cooking herbs have concentrated amounts of phytochemicals that come from various plant and vegetable foods as well as fiber and fruits. These phytochemicals are antioxidants and tend to be chemo-preventative which means they tend to protect the body from developing cancer. Some studies have shown that phytochemicals in fruit may decrease the development of colon, lung, liver, and prostate cancers. Discuss the use of herbs with your healthcare provider and evaluate the modern scientific studies supporting their role in cancer prevention and maintaining optimal health.

Hydration

Water bathes our cells and tissues and is essential to good health. The average male needs about 3.7 liters and the average female about 2.7 liters. Pregnant women should drink about 3 liters and lactating moms need about 3.8 liters. Keep in mind a liter is equal to a quart or 32 ounces which is 4 cups of water. So 2.7 liters is approximately 9 to 10 cups of water. Keep in mind that total water consumption includes water in food, beverages, and drinking water. A recent hydration tip I learned from Fitness Magazine:

Drink half your body weight in ounces

So if you weigh 100 pounds, your daily hydration level should be 50oz. Now, that's a simple easy to remember rule of thumb!

We know that **alcohol** has both healthy and unhealthy effects on our bodies mainly due to the amount of alcohol we consume. So, to better understand how much you might be consuming each week, visit this new website at http://alcoholcontent.gov. Here are the recommendations for low alcohol use or what the CDC considers moderate alcohol intake:

Women – 1 daily serving

Men – up to 2 servings per day

Remember: a serving is **5oz wine or 1.5 oz spirits**

Some of the known benefits of alcohol include:

Heart disease risk reduction about 25%

Raise the good HDL cholesterol

Decrease the risk of dementia and other cognitive impairments

Reduce gallstone formation in women

Lower the risk of diabetes by controlling insulin and triglyceride levels

Women are especially vulnerable to the bad effects of excess alcohol for two reasons. Women have 50% less alcohol dehydrogenase which is an enzyme that metabolizes alcohol in the stomach. So women absorb 100% of the alcohol they drink. Women also have less water and more fat in their bodies so alcohol is more concentrated in their bloodstream.

Alcohol like any other drug should be taken relative to your body size. Smaller and lightweight people need less alcohol to feel relaxed and sociable than heavier and larger people. You can also become physically addicted to alcohol like other drugs. The four classic symptoms to watch are:

Craving – a strong need or urge to drink

Physical dependence – withdrawal symptoms like nausea, sweating, shakiness and anxiety after stopping drinking

Loss of control – not being able to stop drinking once drinking has begun

Tolerance – the need to drink greater amounts to get "high"

If you think alcohol is a problem in your life, speak with your doctor for a definitive diagnosis. There are many treatment options today both inpatient and outpatient facilities, medications, and counseling that can help you recover from this addiction.

Alcohol intake is also a risk factor associated with the following cancers:

Breast

Colon and rectum

Esophagus

Liver

Pancreas

Throat (pharaynx)

Voice box

According to the American Cancer Society (ACS) the risk increases with the amount of alcohol consumed.

No Smoking Ever!

The 2014 Surgeon General Report on Smoking marked the 50th anniversary of the efforts to reduce the effect of smoking on the nation's health. This "winnable" battle has made tremendous strides, but we must continue our efforts with more potent tobacco products and the consequent addiction. This year's report adds to the list of smoking effects on the health of Americans:

Risk factor for 12 cancers: bladder, breast, colorectal, head/neck, liver, lung, pancreatic, prostate, skin, stomach, throat, and uterine.

Causative link for these diseases: diabetes, ectopic pregnancy, male erectile dysfunction, rheumatoid arthritis and some immune function dysfunction.

Since the First Surgeon General Report in 1964, 20 million Americans have died due to smoking. 2.5 million or 12.5% of those were nonsmokers who died from heart disease or lung cancer due to secondhand smoke exposures. Also, 100,000 babies have died due to complications of maternal smoking including SIDS, prematurity, and low birth weight. The 2006 Surgeon General Report provided evidence that there is no safe level of exposure to secondhand smoke. Although the **rate of smoking has decreased from 42% in 1964 to 19% today**, the products are more potent in terms of carcinogenic potential. Today's smokers have a much higher risk for lung cancer, and chronic obstructive pulmonary (COPD) than smokers in 1964.

Three diet culprits: fat, salt, and sugar

The single most important concept for healthy nutrition is a balanced diet. We all know that the three culprits, salt, fat, and sugar, can damage our health when consumed in an unhealthy amount each day.

Too much salt in our diet increases our risk for high blood pressure, kidney damage, and heart disease.

Too much sugar increases our risk of weight gain, tooth decay, and high triglycerides which can lead to heart disease.

Too much unhealthy fats in our diet increases our risk for diabetes, heart disease, and cancer.

So, here is your daily RDAs for Sugar, Fat, and Salt

Salt **RDA:**   **2300mg/day** for most adults

Fat RDA is relative to your caloric intake.

> **1500 calories require 33-58 gms fat**
>
> **2000 calories requires 44-78 gms of fat**
>
> **2500 calories requires 56-97 gm fat.**

Sugar RDA is **6 tsp (24gm) daily for adult women** and **9 tsp for adult men (36gms).**

Use this information to compare the nutrition information on fast foods and you will easily understand why these food choices can rob you of a daily dose of sugar, fat and salt in one serving. I recently switched my Greek yogurt brand to consume less sugar. Remember each teaspoon of sugar contains 4 grams of sugar. So, read your labels carefully and make smart nutrition choices each day.

The Role of Registered Dieticians

Seek the advice of a professional registered dietician to provide you with a personalized nutrition program to meet your specific health needs or chronic disease. Registered dietician can also assist people in various life stages such as pregnancy, growing years, and old age, as well as food allergies, living with chronic diseases, and recovery from surgery and chemotherapy.

Part III: A is for Activity/Exercise in your RNA Action Plan

We discussed earlier the American Heart Association (AHA) recommendation for ideal exercise as 150 minutes per week or 30 minutes of aerobic activity 5 times per week or 75 minutes of moderate duration. Check with your doctor to determine the appropriate heartbeat threshold for you and the appropriate level of intensity for you.

The American Sport and Health Foundation and Human Performance (HP) Institute employs science-based information and an interdisciplinary approach to increase human energy and enhance human performance. Their recent studies found that **our energy level not our time management is what keeps us from exercising often.** Yet, Americans refuse to believe the counterintuitive truth - when we exercise for short periods of time, we actually gain energy and focus.

The human energy pyramid consists of four levels:

Physical: higher energy fitness, frequent exercise

Emotional: sustained levels of confidence, positive feelings and resilience

Mental: Increased mental alertness, focus and preparation for work

Spiritual: Higher feelings of being fully engaged with work and personal life

This is the exercise equivalent of Maslow's Hierarchy of Human Needs for Quality of life!

Only about **20% of Americans actually get the recommended weekly amount of physical activity**. More recent research suggests the even brief intervals or so called 'microbursts' of high intensity workouts can achieve results. One example is the 7 minute workout that can be completed two or three times a day.

A recent article probed the answer to the question: what is more to blame for the obesity epidemic – lack of exercise or eating too much? The published study in the July 7 American *Journal of Medicine* discovered that over the past 20 years the **rate of no exercise was**:

52% of U.S. women and 44% of US men

During the same time period, the average **BMI (body mass index) rose from an average of 18 to 39!** Overall caloric intake did not change. Stanford University researchers also measured abdominal obesity, a marker for mortality in people with average BMI levels.

Abdominal obesity is defined as a waist circumference of:

34.65 inches or more for women

40.16 inches or more for men

So efforts to curb obesity must stress daily physical activity and exercise.

Here are some easy facts to ponder about walking:

Walkers live longer, weigh less, have lower blood pressure, and enjoy better health

Just 30 minutes of walking a day can prevent type 2 diabetes.

Walking a mile or more per day cuts your risk of death from all causes in half

Walking 5-9 miles per week lowers your risk of memory loss and improves bone density

Walking 12.5 miles a week or more cuts the risk of stroke 50%.

Just 30 minutes a day of walking reduces feelings of tension and depression and burns 7 pounds a year

A brisk 45 minute morning walk improves sleep significantly and reduces insomnia.

Women who walk briskly 3 or more hours per week reduce their heart disease level by 30-40% and men cut their risk by 50%

So, let's all get walking. It is a no-brainer!!

Prevention Magazine shared the results of a recent University of Virginia study by an exercise physiologist that looked at men and women completing **fifteen 10-minute exercise routines a week.** That is equivalent of about 20 minutes of mild to moderate exercise per day as recommended by the American Heart Association. **After only 21 days, the aerobic fitness of the participants was equal to that of people up to 15 years younger. Their strength, muscle endurance, and flexibility were equal to people 20 years younger**. So, yes small exercise periods pay back huge dividends for your longevity and quality of life!

Here are 10 suggestions for short bursts of exercise:

A 5-minute power walk up and 5 minute walk down your street

Exercise on a treadmill when a sick loved one is napping

2 five minute intervals of jumping jacks or stretching exercises

Jog in place when commercials interrupt your favorite TV show

Do leg exercises and lifts with small weights at work or when you watch TV

Use the stairs and walk the airport concourse when you travel

Do calf stretches at work riding in elevators

Take work or lunch breaks climbing stairs for 5-10 minutes

Walk to work or take a walk during your lunch break

Stop twice a day on long car trips to take a brisk walk

Healthy Numbers to Remember for a Longer Life

2 hours of TV a day. More hours increase your triglyceride level and decrease your HDL or good cholesterol level

7 or more servings a day of fruits and vegetables reduces risk of death by 42% according to a recent British study

7 hours of sleep a day controls your weight. 50% of people who sleep less than 5 hours a night are obese

Keep your commute to 20 miles R/T. Longer commutes increase blood pressure and chornic stress and worry

1:2 is the healthiest ratio of your waist:height. Thicker waists can lead to metabolic syndrome.

Importance of Strength Training

The Mayo Clinic describes strength training as an important part of an overall fitness program. Did you realize that strength training reduces body fat, increases lean muscle mass, and burns calories? Muscle mass decreases with age so strength training gives the added advantage of preserving muscle mass at any age. Its other benefits include building strong bones by increasing bone density, tones your muscles so it is easier to lose weight, build your stamina and balance, and reduce the signs and symptoms of chronic conditions like back pain, arthritis, obesity, heart disease, and diabetes. Finally, regular strength training improves attention especially in older adults according to recent research.

There is a wide variety of options to engage in strength training. You can do pushups, abdominal crunches, and leg squats. Or you can use resistance tubing which you stretch to provide resistance training. Classic barbells and dumbbells are free weights to consider as well. Finally, weight machines are offered at many fitness centers and you can purchase for home use.

It is important to consult your healthcare professional about what type of strength training is the best fit for you. Listen to your body, get proper instructions on the use of weight training equipment, and rest your muscles at least one full day between workouts to prevent injury. Two or three strength training sessions per week of 15-30 minutes is usually sufficient.

Noticeable improvements in strength and stamina usually occur in a few weeks. Many strength training enthusiasts and trainers notice a faster metabolic rate which improves weight loss.

Stretching for Health

Stretching for health and fitness is part of an overall physical activity program. Stretching improves our range of motion in our joints and decreases the risk of injuries when exercising. The improved flexibility by stretching our joints, muscles, and tendons makes them stronger and less prone to injury by increasing blood flow to these areas.

Proper technique to stretch effectively and safely is essential. Bad technique can lead to injury. Here are some general rules to follow:

Stretch after you exercise when your muscles are warmed up

Focus on major muscle groups like your calves, thighs, hips, lower back, neck and shoulders. Be sure to stretch both sides equally and don't bounce, but stretch smoothly.

Hold your stretches for about 30 seconds breathing normally as you stretch. If you have problem areas, holding longer stretches for 50-60 seconds may be beneficial.

Expect tension in your muscles as you stretch but not pain. If it hurts, you are pushing too far. Hold the stretch in the position where you just feel tension.

Tailor stretches to your sport or everyday activities. Office workers may want to stretch neck, shoulder, and lower back muscles to reduce tension from prolonged sitting.

You can achieve the best results by stretching regularly, at least 2-3 times per week. If you don't stretch regularly, you will lose the flexibility and range of motion benefits.

Interject movement into your stretches such as yoga or tai chi which increases your flexibility.

Stretching won't prevent overuse injuries. Talk to your doctor or physical therapist about how best to personalize your stretches to cope with your health concern.

Balance Exercises

Evidenced based studies have revealed that balance exercises can prevent falls in people with low bone density and osteoporosis. These are simple exercises that usually don't require special equipment or a great amount of time. Some examples are Tai Chi and Yoga positions, balancing on one foot with arms outstretched or in the meditation prayer position for 60 seconds. Some newer medical research findings are looking more closely at the balance test as a possible way to diagnose brain vascular problems earlier.

Interval Training

Variety and novelty is important to the body and the brain as we learned earlier in Chapter 3. So, after establishing a regular exercise schedule, break it up about once a week with a new twist. For instance, you can alternate a slow walk pace with a faster pace for a few minutes. This extra challenge can raise your level of fitness. Be sure to enlist the advice of certified training professionals when altering your usual exercise routine and always listen to your body.

Chapter 3: Health Challenge Goal

I challenge you to learn the 4-7-8 deep breathing method.

Chapter 4 - The Prevention Core: Managing Your Health Risks

Education is a powerful predictor of longer life spans.

Education exerts its direct beneficial effects on health through the adoption of healthier lifestyles, better ability to cope with stress, and more effective management of chronic diseases.

Health Affairs 2014 study

The past chapter summarized the holistic view of health from a prevention based healthcare system perspective. We learned how to take care of our body and mind with healthy habits. We learned about the three equal legs of the health triangle: rest/ nutrition/activity.

Prevention has two parts: primary and secondary. Primary prevention is aimed at healthy habits that prevent chronic disease development. These habits promote your good health and wellness and keep your biometrics in a healthy range. Your RNA plan is an example of primary prevention. Epidemiologic study findings that identify occupational risk factors associated with certain cancers are another example. The goal of secondary prevention is to screen and diagnose chronic conditions especially in "at risk" people. These efforts include screening tests and procedures to discover unknown risk factors and also monitor known risk factors. Secondary prevention also prevents the progression of a disease to a later stage and prevent complications from the disease.

Take Charge of Your Health

This chapter introduces a three step plan to take charge of your health today. Step One discusses the need to create a personalized RNA plan to maximize your health and wellness and maintain healthy biometrics. Step Two describes how you identify your own health risk factors and find ways to minimize their potential negative influence on your health. Step Three examines how you manage and treat any controllable risk factor that threatens your good health.

Step One: Your Personalized Healthcare-Equalizer RNA Action Plan

The previous chapter emphasized the need to develop an RNA Action Plan to take charge of your health and wellness goals. Your physical exam visit is the perfect opportunity to share your health and wellness goals with your health provider and document a measurement goal and target deadline to achieve it. For instance, your Rest goal might be to get at least 7 hours of sleep each night. After using the BBC sleep profiler, I discovered that I am best served by my "early to bed early to rise" circadian rhythm. It is important to understand how your body works and stick to what works. Avoid things that disrupt your sleep like bedtime snacks and drinks, bedtime worries, and restless bodies that need to relax before slumber. Be sure to notice how you feel and act when you are well rested.

Don't forget that R also stands for daily relaxation. So, pick and choose your favorite relaxation exercise or de-stressor activity and schedule time for it daily.

Your Nutrition goal can be quite simple like eat a serving of a fruit and/or vegetable with each meal. Eat seasonal fresh fruits and vegetables that you can eat raw so there is no preparation time. Once you are successful with increasing your fruits and vegetable intake, you can carry a water bottle to hydrate yourself. The simple rule of half your weight in ounces makes it easy. Other changes like adopting more plant based foods, decreasing saturated red meats, and adding fiber may take longer and may disrupt your digestive system. Keeping a food diary may be helpful. Remember, slowly changing your diet is always best. Listen to what your body tells you about different foods and how those foods affect your digestive system. A visit with a registered dietician can be very helpful in designing healthy food preparation methods as well as sample menu plans to try. As you get comfortable with your balanced diet, be sure to measure your daily sugar, fat, and salt by reading your food labels. You may discover that one serving of your favorite fast food exceeds your daily intake of all three! Maybe it is time to get a replacement comfort food!!

Your activity level is probably the most difficult for most people to adopt as recent studies indicate. However, short periods of activity can be very helpful. So, start small and reward yourself for success. Again, notice your moods, your strength, your energy level, and how your clothes fit as you increase your daily activity level. Pick a biometric you and your healthcare provider want to monitor and measure it once a week to see if it improves. Find the best activity level that you can sustain each day. Alternate your activities such as stretching, walking, and balance exercises to break the monotony and keep it interesting. Make plans for how you will stay active while on vacation or visiting friends and family over the holidays.

Changing our daily habits can be quite challenging. Statistics and knowledge can help identify what bad lifestyle habits we have and what the deleterious effect it has on our present and future health. However, motivating us to change and making the change in our habits is where we fail to launch successful new habits. So, let's look at how long and how to change our habits successfully.

A recent Wall Street Journal article cited a 2009 study by University College London researchers that arrived at the conclusion that it takes **66 days to form a habit**. Having a specific goal is most helpful. By creating an action plan with the goal, you will be more successful. The action plan specifies the when, where and how the activity will take place. This new wave thinking assumes that situations trigger our actions. Stanford University researchers found that regular exercisers who received calls about physical activity were more likely to be exercising regularly six months later.

Now, a recent Parade article on breaking bad habits by Gretchen Rubin, author of the book **Better Than Before: Mastering the Habits of Our Everyday Lives**, proposes a fascinating theory. Rubin has developed 4 personality categories and says the trick is to tailor your habits to suit your personality. The **Upholder** personality meets outer and inner expectations and usually forms new habits easily because she responds well to other people's as well as her own deadlines. The **Questioner** resists outer expectations and seeks to meet inner expectations. This personality type will only change a habit if it makes sense to them. **Obligers** meet outer expectations and resist meeting their inner expectations. This personality type works hard to meet other's expectations, but may end up disappointing themselves. **Rebels** resent and resist habits because they resist inner and outer expectations.

Rubin recommends clarifying your habit with specific actions such as packing a daily lunch instead of eating fast food. One helpful suggestion is measure your food intake with a food diary or a food tracker app. When it comes to exercise, pairing a desirable activity with a new unfavorable activity can sometimes work. For instance, each morning after I drink my jasmine green tea, I put on my athletic shoes and jump on the treadmill. The **Obliger** might think she has no time for exercise. Maybe she can find 5 minute exercise sessions during work breaks and a 30 minutes brisk walk on her lunch hour with a co-worker.

The **Questioner** needs to find the right reason to motivate himself to exercise. The **Rebel** may benefit from mindfulness techniques that focus on making a conscious decision to become healthy. Rebels feel success when they are in control of their decisions. So, distracting themselves with 4-7-8 relaxation breaths, reading emails, and taking green-scape breaks may give them the courage to say no to that glass of wine, fast food choice, or candy bar.

So, learn to reward your hard work with treats that are healthy for you. However, the ultimate reward is the freedom you get from self-control and constant decisions to change the bad habit. Once you succeed, the less you have to drain your willpower. This growth within our self leads to true happiness.

You may find the consumer brochures recently released by the Agency for Healthcare Research and Quality (AHRQ) in 2014 entitled, *Stay Healthy.* The brochures give information on tips for good health and preventive care and various screening guidelines. The information uses evidenced based healthcare recommendations developed by the U.S. Preventive Services Task Force. Learn more about his agency as well as AHRQ in the next chapter on Finding Quality Healthcare Information. There are four brochures.

Here is the link www.ahrq.gov.

Men: Stay Healthy at Any Age

Men: Stay Healthy at 50+

Women: Stay Healthy at Any Age

Women: Stay Healthy at 50+

Let your RNA plan be a work in progress as you meet one goal and then set a new one. You decide what healthy habits you want to adopt and then measure your progress. You can improve your quality of life and may even decrease some of your medications for chronic conditions as you improve your daily healthy habits. With the money you save, take a trip or visit a favorite museum or restaurant or save it for your long retirement!

.

Step Two: Personalized Risk Management

Good health is really about risk management. Usually in medicine, we like to follow the rules of cause and effect. I learned valuable lessons in my Epidemiology course in graduate school. An agent is known to cause a disease if it is always present for the effect to occur. For instance, you need exposure to the flu virus, to get influenza symptoms. When a specific cause is consistently linked with a specific effect, there is little uncertainty about the diagnosis, and intervention is always warranted. These evidenced based interventions are common in control of such communicable diseases as the HIV virus as the cause of AIDS and the polio virus causing poliomyelitis.

However, with cancer and other chronic diseases, determining the cause is more complicated because exposure doesn't immediately cause the disease. This latency period makes it difficult to precisely determine the cause. When there is no direct cause and effect relationship, but an association between the two, those agents are called **risk factors**.

According to the American Cancer Society, 1 million people get cancer each year. Body weight has the strongest evidence linked to cancer. Excess body weight contributes to 1 out of 5 or 20% of all cancer deaths. **Obesity** is clearly linked to the following cancers:

Breast (esp. postmenopausal)

Colon and Rectum

Endometrium (uterine)

Esophagus

Kidney

Pancreas

Obesity is a likely cause of the following cancers:

Cervix

Gallbladder

Liver

Non-Hodgkins Lymphoma

Multiple Myeloma

Ovary

(Aggressive) Prostate Cancers

As we learned in the past chapter, smoking also elevates your cancer risk so the synergistic effect of smoking and obesity tip the scale for your increased cancer risk. The American Cancer Society lists the current **risk factors for cancer as:**

> **Alcohol consumption**
>
> **Environmental/chemical exposures**
>
> **Excess body weight**
>
> **Inactivity**
>
> **Radiation exposure**
>
> **Smoking**

Risk factors have become the early intervention point to prevent a chronic disease. They are also the endpoint to controlling the symptoms of that disease and preventing serious complications from it. So risk factors are important to identify and minimize if possible. It is important to identify some of your risk factors by carefully documenting and verifying family medical history records as well as considering DNA and genetic testing. We are now discovering genetic factors associated with some cancers and other diseases.

Accurate Family History

Compiling an accurate family medical history is your top priority to take charge of your health. If you know what diseases your family members had or their cause of death, you can take steps to prevent or reduce your risk. Research has indicated that family medical history is an efficient and accurate tool for assessing disease risk. A recent study in the *Journal of the National Cancer Institute* demonstrates, however, that a cancer patient's accuracy in reporting the cancer diagnosis of their relatives was low to moderate. Inaccurate histories may result in unnecessary screenings.

Your **family history should span three generations.** Start with your parents, siblings and children and span outward to include your grandparents, aunts and uncles, as well as nieces, nephews, and grandchildren and then your cousins. It is important to **document the cause of death and age of mortality**. Some genetic cancers usually strike before age 50.

Lifestyle information is also helpful such as diet, exercise habits, smoking and alcohol use.

Here are some resources to consider:

My Family Health Portrait online at
https://familyhistory.hhs.gov

CDC Public Health Genomics website
(www.cdc.gov/genomics/famhistory)

The American Society of Human Genetics
(talkhealthhistory.org)

Hereditary Cancer and Other Genetic Risk Assessment

Hereditary Cancer risk is important to assess accurately.
Cancer that occurs before age 50 in any individual or
family member tends to be a sign of a hereditary cancer.
Multiple cases of cancer in your personal or family history
also raise a red flag to a possible hereditary cancer. The
risk of hereditary cancer can be passed down through
generations on both sides of the family.

Are there early, multiple or rare breast cancers in your
family? You may be at increased cancer risk and may need
a personalized screening recommendation

Are there early, multiple or rare colon cancers in the family? If so, you may need a personalized screening regimen that you and your healthcare provider can develop.

It is important to understand what cancer metastasis really means. Many cancers travel away from their primary organ and metastasize to a distant organ such as the brain, lung, liver, or the bones. When this occurs, the patient is told they have metastasized breast cancer or lung cancer. Some people mistakenly think the patient has a new cancer such as liver cancer or brain cancer in addition to the primary site cancer. So, be careful when you do family histories and examine cause of death. Be sure you know the primary cancer site to record.

Genetic Testing and Screening

Our DNA is what makes us human and unique. The sequence of our DNA as well as the specific gene and gene markers that we inherit can influence our risk for various diseases and conditions. DNA sequencing companies are now discovering that genes also influence how we metabolize drugs and foods and interact with our environment. So, let's embrace the need for genetic testing for ourselves to learn more about our health risks and understand how to prevent, treat, and cure cancers. Let us also seek to understand the DNA of our health enemies: bacteria, cancer, diabetes, etc. Groundbreaking research is unraveling novel and creative ways to stop disabling and deadly diseases by analyzing the DNA of the offending agent. This knowledge can stop the growth of the disease and limit the damage to our body. Truly, this is the immune system defending itself against these invaders. The great advantage these DNA tests and treatments bring is less damage to surrounding parts of the body including our immune system. This is the future of personalized healthcare and treatment!

Dr. Eric Topol, a Genomics Professor at Scripps Research Institute, has coined the term, "molecular stethoscope" for the next 200 years to describe the clinical applications resulting from NIH's human genome project. The "alien" DNA found in healthy individuals can be tested for specific genetic mutations. Today, pregnant women can now submit a blood sample instead of the invasive and sometimes dangerous amniocentesis procedure for DNA sequencing. Thanks to Dr. Stephen Quake, Stanford University Professor of Bioengineering and Applied Physics, we can now detect these fetal chromosomal abnormalities in blood and a new test for early signs of organ rejection in transplant recipients by measuring levels of donor DNA. Alien DNA can now be sequenced to diagnose the source of a nonspecific infection in patients where blood cultures have failed to identify the infectious agent. The alien DNA tests can also detect genetic mutations that are driving particular cancers and can help select appropriate personalized treatments that will work.

Genetic evaluations and counseling sessions can help clarify and quantify risk reductions that can successfully reduce your risk for certain hereditary cancers and other conditions. For instance, hereditary breast cancer can sometimes be reduced by as much as 53% using Tamoxifen, up to 68% with prophylactic mastectomy and up to 96% with removal of the ovaries. Ovarian cancer risk can be mitigated by as much as 60% with oral contraceptives and up to 96% with surgery to remove the ovaries. So, pursue genetic testing and the advice of trained genetics counselors to build a personalized risk reduction plan for yourself and your loved ones.

Communicable Disease Prevention

As you read earlier, much of our communicable disease control efforts are focused on known causes. The annual flu immunization campaigns have decreased the death rate and disability from serious influenza epidemics. Immunizations are a lifetime commitment. The CDC immunization schedules mentioned in the next chapter give the current recommendations for both adults and children. Discuss with your health provider your personalized need for certain extra immunizations like the shingles vaccine, pneumonia vaccine and Hepatitis B and C vaccines recently developed. Also, when you travel, you may sometimes be asked to get additional vaccines to prevent you from contracting a communicable disease prevalent in the area you are visiting. The CDC and State Department websites are helpful in identifying the health requirements for travel to certain countries. So checkout their website before you travel abroad.

Screening Guidelines

In a prevention model of care, risk appraisal calculations are usually followed by recommendations for various screening tests and procedures. In the US, the same principles are used to evaluate the benefits of a screening test or a drug or a treatment protocol. Smart consumers frequently read research study results that report on the relative risk of a stated test or treatment or drug. We assume that these risk measurements are definitive and are based on unequivocal evidence which leads to an "illusion of certainty."

Unfortunately, consumers forget that there is an element of uncertainty which is built into the assessment process for determining health benefits and risks. The National Research Council has an accepted risk assessment paradigm as an analytic technique to assess risk for the scientific, regulatory, and medical communities. Risk assessment presents a way to navigate "iffy" decisions when cause and effect can't yet be proven. Risk is simply a possibility. Unfortunately, this level of uncertainty also poses a limitation on the usefulness of such data.

In the book, **The Illusion of Certainty,** the environmental science authors, Eric Rifkin and Edward Bouwer, explain how consumers need to face critical questions about how risk is calculated for an individual. It is important to discriminate between population based risk guidelines that are meant for communities. Consumers need to be careful how their personal risk is evaluated and measured.

The authors explain the difference between two popular risk assessment tools that are commonly used in many screening and new drug/test studies. The first risk assessment measurement tool is the **absolute risk or ARR**.

This represents your **personal risk of developing a disease over a specified period of time**. This measurement is frequently used in chronic disease research, but these numbers are **rarely provided to the public.** The second risk measurement method is the **Relative Risk Reduction (RRR)** rate. This is employed by pharmaceutical and medical device makers in their studies to compare the risk in a control group and an experimental group. These studies are often done to show the public the benefit of a new drug or screening test. However, the **RRR can sometimes overestimate the true individual risk** since it compares the relative risk for a community not an individual. So, applying the study results to your own risk assessment is the tricky part!

A recent review by two career scientists spoke out against financial incentives within drug research studies and how they harm patients. Their critique was published in the journal, *Expert Review of Clinical Pharmacology.* The pair analyzed the data in various statin trials and reached the conclusion that the statin advocates had used "statistical deception" to create the illusion that statins were "wonder drugs" and disregarded their significant adverse effects. The **absolute risk** is the effect of the drug on a single person. Their studies indicate the absolute risk was actually **1% meaning only one in 100 people taking the drug will**

have one less heart attack. The statin advocate researchers however transformed that 1% effect using the **"relative risk" statistic** creating the impression that **30-50% of people would benefit from using the drug.** Their error was using the relative risk incorrectly and representing that as the absolute risk for an individual.

The adverse effects of statins include increased rates of cancer, cataracts, diabetes, cognitive impairments, and musculoskeletal disorders. One long-term study demonstrated a dramatic increase in the incidence of breast cancer in women using statins for more than 10 years. The statin trials were usually terminated within 2 to 5 years - a period too short to see most cancers develop. This study illustrates the need for the public to be wary of conflicts of interest in the medical community and pharmaceutical industry. The editor of the main British Medical Journal responded to this article by demanding drug companies to release all of their records on undisclosed adverse effects of statins in their clinical trials. This journal also introduced a new standard for any article published – they will be authored by experts without financial ties to industry. Perhaps American medical journals can learn from this precedent.

You can now see that when mortality rates are very low as in this study, the ARR becomes smaller and RRR remains constant. Thus the **RRR enhances the risk and makes it seem more dramatic. It also tends to overestimate the benefit of the new drug or test.** So you can see how this rate is popular with medical device makers and pharmaceutical studies. Our job as smart consumers is to critically examine the new research study findings with dramatic improvements. Find out what risk measurement technique was used, the funding source, and ask about side effects of long-term use of the drug.

The merit of screening tests and procedures is now under the medical microscope for many reasons. Now we have long-term clinical trial data to examine the effectiveness of screening tests and procedures. We have data that demonstrate patient harm in the form of unnecessary biopsies, false positive findings, and complications from the test procedure itself. These have not been fully appreciated and researched in the past. Screening programs are evolving and changing based on new evidence. The American Cancer Society has now adopted new guidelines using evidenced based data that is contrary to old guidelines. Some of these changes include:

Prostate cancer screenings are now not routine but rather a discussion with your PCP

Breast cancer screening frequency differs by your age and risk factors

This movement is a positive one and emphasizes the need to for consumers to develop   personalized screening recommendation with your provider. Community screening measures are commonly used to decrease the incidence of many serious life threatening diseases like cancer. They educate the public about the silent nature of certain diseases, identify first symptoms and seek to identify people at increased risk. Two examples are women with dense breasts and patients who develop colon polyps. You can't control these risk factors, but screening tests can measure and monitor these risk factors.

You can control other risk factors for many chronic conditions like smoking, poor fruit and vegetable intake, inactivity, and high alcohol intake and thereby reduce your overall risk for the condition. Risk management is merely a math problem where you reduce the risks you can control and participate in screening programs to control risk factors you can't control.

In Chapter 5, you will learn about a physician initiative to warn patients about unnecessary tests and procedures unless you are at high risk. It is very important that you discuss your personal and family history risks for certain diseases with your doctor so a personalized screening guideline can be developed.

Step Three: Personalized Chronic Disease Action Plan

The stoplight approach to asthma control was developed while I worked at the Asthma and Allergy Foundation of America (AAFA). This written blueprint gave patients an action plan that prescribed future actions to take based on measurements of a certain biometric, peak flow meter readings. This personal radar system or biofeedback approach helps patients get acquainted with how their body feels when their chronic disease is not well controlled and when it is.

The **green zone** is the **healthy zone** which is 85-100% of peak flow rates for asthmatics. Usually this is your routine care – medications, environmental control measures, nutrition suggestions, as well as exercise and sleep habits to follow to control your disease or risk factor or biometric. Decide with your healthcare provider what biometric you need to measure for your chronic condition.

Yellow zone is the **caution zone**. With asthmatics, the yellow zone is when the peak flow measurement is between 50-84%. Detecting these early changes in breathing capacity assists the patient in diagnosing the need for additional medications to stop these fluctuations and return to green zone peak flow meter readings. Your action or treatment plan will identity what medications or actions to follow to keep your prescribed biometric in this 50-84% zone.

Red zone is the **emergency zone.** For asthmatics, this is peak flow meter readings below 50%. This zone necessitates emergency or urgent medical attention. Find out from your healthcare provider what biometric measurement above or below the 50% level or which specific symptoms need emergency or urgent attention.

This asthma action plan can be applied to the self-management of other chronic diseases like diabetes, high blood pressure, kidney disease, and heart disease. This action plan approach produces an educated and engaged consumer and a responsive healthcare team. Patients learn good detective skills to monitor subtle changes in a selected biometric measurement as indicated by the use of special meters and tests at home. This monitoring is imperative to achieve maximum control of your disease and limit complications. This written blueprint facilitates important data communication with your healthcare team to prevent emergency room admissions and hospitalizations. So, design a chronic disease action plan with your provider and keep a copy for yourself at home.

Chapter 4: Health Challenge Goal: I challenge you to share your Chronic Disease Plan or RNA Plan with your doctor at your next checkup visit. Remember to make goals clear, specific, and measurable.

Chapter 5: Quality Health Care Information

Knowledge is power.

Francis Bacon

Each man judges well the things he knows.

Aristotle

Knowledge is power and it helps us become smart shoppers of quality healthcare services. This keeps us healthy. We need a wide variety of healthcare information today. This list includes healthy habits, prevention, diagnosis and treatment recommendations, screening guidelines, and performance metrics to judge the quality and safety of healthcare services by providers and facilities. Our information sources need to be evidenced based, independent of commercial interests, and current.

The use of evidenced based recommendations for prevention, diagnosis and treatment has traditionally been provided by clinical trials, the gold standard, in the scientific community. These large trials usually have large sample sizes, an experimental as well as a control group, and examine any confounding factors that could also explain the results. The long-term Nurses Study and the Framingham Heart Study, are treasure troves of data that examine healthcare outcomes over many years. These studies have been valuable in measuring the impact of various diet, exercise, and medication habits of these populations over time and have the additional benefit of large sample sizes. The medical and scientific community has always looked to national and international clinical trials to replicate and validate earlier findings before definitive and new evidenced based guidelines and recommendations are issued.

The Consumer Bible for Quality Prevention Information: USPSTF

The US Preventive Services Task Force (USPSTF) was created in 1984 as an independent group of national experts in prevention and evidence-based medicine assigned to improve the health of all Americans by creating evidence-based recommendations about clinical preventive services. These services might include screening, counseling or preventive medications. The USPSTF is composed of volunteer practicing clinicians from various disciplines – internal medicine, family medicine, pediatrics, behavioral health, obstetrics/gynecology, and nursing.

When USPSTF was established in 1984, Congress required the Department of Health and Human Services or HHS to support the task forces' work. The 1998 Public Health Service Act and the 2010 Patient Protection and Affordable Care Act designated the Agency for Healthcare Research and Quality (**AHRQ**) to provide administrative, research, technical and communication support to the Task Force.

Accordingly, the Director of AHRQ appoints new USPSTF members with guidance from the Chair of the Task Force. However, it is important to know that the Task Force is an independent body and its work and recommendations do not require AHRQ or HHS approval.

Go to http://USPreventiveServicesTaskForce.org and see the latest complete USPSTF recommendation statements along with the supporting scientific evidence. Over the years the recommendations have been adopted by individual health care providers, professional organizations, integrated health systems, health plans and insurers, and public programs, such as Centers for Medicare and Medicaid Services (CMS), health quality metric groups and national health objectives like the Healthy Peoples Report. **Now the recommendations are considered by many to be definitive standards for preventive services. These evidenced based findings with letter grades attached to them indicate the level of scientific confidence behind the new guideline. The USPSTF strives to evaluate evidence free from the influence of politics, special interests, and advocacy.** The work of this task force is central to the preventive benefits covered under the Patient Protection and Affordable Care Act of 2010.

AHCQ has released its Prevention brochures for 2014 – get your free copy at www.ahrq.gov website and download yours today. This agency also helps consumers find a Medical Home practice group in their community that has achieved this quality designation. Read more about this in Chapter 6. This agency also houses the **Patient Centered Outcomes Research Institute (PCORI)** created with the implementation of the ACA that read about in Chapter 2. This Center is an excellent example of how our healthcare system can become more accountable for effective and efficient services by continuous improvement. This is value and science driven healthcare of the future. Visit the PCORI and evaluate their Clinical Effectiveness Research (CER) trials and results on various diseases and conditions as well as healthcare delivery practice changes.

CDC: Our Tax Dollars at work!

The 60 year old Centers for Disease Control agency works 24/7 to protect America's public health from both domestic and foreign health threats. The CDC promotes quality of life through the prevention and control of disease, injury, and disability. It is committed to programs that reduce the health and economic consequences of our leading causes of death and disability.

Visit www.cdc.gov and find the following helpful information:

Alphabetized index of diseases and conditions

Annual vaccine and immunization schedule for children and adults

Healthy Living Recommendations

Injury, Violence and Safety Prevention Tips

Environmental Health Concerns

Workplace Safety and Health

Traveler's Health and Vaccinations

BMI Calculator

Emergency Preparedness

The CDC also publishes fact sheets explaining how this agency works to protect you, your family, friends and communities. The CDC team includes researchers, scientists, doctors, nurses, economists, communicators, educators, technologists, and epidemiologists. The CDC website is your go to place for information about influenza, community acquired infections like MRSA and C Diff, as

well as West Nile Virus, Ebola, and other public health
threats.

Quality Diagnostic and Treatment information

Once you develop symptoms of a chronic disease or have
been diagnosed with a new disease or condition, you need
information to properly diagnose the condition and find
effective and recommended treatments. The National
Institutes of Health, NIH, has always been viewed as the
premier medical research agency in the United States.

According to their website, www.NIH.gov, this government
agency supports scientific studies that turn discovery into
health. The NIH mission is to seek fundamental knowledge
about the nature and behavior of living systems and then
apply that knowledge to enhance life and longevity by
reducing illness and disability. The National Institutes of
Health also promotes the highest level of scientific
integrity, public accountability, and social responsibility in
the conduct of science. It strives to research the causes,
diagnosis, prevention, and cure for human diseases. Its
research efforts also investigate human growth and
development, biologic effects of environmental

contaminants, and understanding mental, addictive, and physical disorders.

Clinical trials are the research method that NIH employs to research our nation's health concerns. This type of clinical research is at the heart of medical advances. Clinical trials explore new ways to prevent, detect and treat disease. Their goal is to determine if a new test or treatment works and is safe. Some trials explore improving quality care for people with chronic diseases. These trials recruit both healthy volunteers as well as disease sufferers for participation. They are usually conducted in three phases: Phase I sets parameters for whether the new test is effective; Phase II determines the appropriate patients that can most benefit; and Phase III sets the safest, effective dose that minimizes patient harm.

Learn more about clinical trials and these other topics by visiting the National Institutes of Health website:

Talking to Your Doctor

Clinical Trials and You

Healthfinder.gov is a health information list of phone numbers for helpful information on various diseases

Health Services locator to find physicians, dentists and other providers in your area

Visit www.PubMed.gov is also part of the NIH network of services. This wonderful National Library of Medicine resource can bring the consumer close to both national and international study results including clinical trials. I still remember combing through the stacks in this prestigious medical library in the 1970s to stay abreast of current medical and nursing research results published in professional journals. Now, you can do the same thing from the comfort of home!

I encourage consumers to checkout this excellent resource for finding quality medical research. Here you will also find national and international medical research articles and clinical trial research results including National Registry studies and the famous UK Cochrane Study Review trials.

The Cochrane Library is an independent source of high quality evidence for health care decisions. The Cochrane Central Register of Controlled Trials (CENTRAL) is part of the Cochrane Database of Systematic Review (CDSR) for practitioners and researchers to systematically review the results of randomized clinical trials over a certain time period. Many times this reassessment requires a new look at old data in reference to newer medical research findings from anywhere in the world. This rigorous review process helps insure that medical research findings are constantly updated and revised.

After researching your health condition or disease on the www.pubmed.gov website, you can choose to email or print the free study results abstract. If you desire the full published study article, it will direct you to the appropriate journal website. Sometimes you can pay for a single article and sometimes you need to be a member of the journal audience to get a copy. Otherwise you always have the option to write down the full study citation from the abstract. Check with your local public library for online partnership access with some medical library search engines.

The National Center for Complementary and Alternative Medicine (NCCAM)

This is the lead government agency for scientific research on complementary and alternative medicine (CAM). They are one of the 27 Institutes of Health within the HHS or Department of Health and Human Services. The mission of NCCAM is to define the usefulness and safety of complementary and alternative medicine interventions through rigorous scientific investigation. This scientific evidence informs decisions by consumers, health care professionals and health policy makers regarding the integration of complementary and alternative medicine.

Visit www.NCCAM.gov for information on the following common complementary and alternative medicine topics:

Acupuncture and acupressure

Massage therapy

Magnet Therapy

Meditation

Supplements

Financial Transparency

Protecting the objectivity and scientific integrity of these research findings has been challenged lately by undue financial influence from funding sources like pharmaceutical and medical device companies as well as payments accepted by physician and scientists. The impartiality of the results has come into question as you read in the last chapter. This is a significant problem since important health policy and treatment decisions are based on new findings about drugs or devices that appear to offer important and sometimes dramatic benefits. In Chapter 8, you will learn more about the various types of financial transparency available to smart healthcare consumers so you can make informed and wise decisions.

A problem has emerged. Can we keep the financial incentives for these large and lucrative trials for pharmaceuticals, medical device makers, and other interest groups from tainting our reported results? As you learned in the previous chapter, statistics can be altered to provide the most compelling and lucrative result to prevail. New treatment diagnosis and treatment guidelines are decided often after reviewing the large clinical trial results. We need to ensure that evidenced based results with significant financial strings are not creating perverse incentives for bad care and unwanted care and expensive care. Smart consumers in this new frontier in healthcare must look carefully for financial disclosure statements after reviewing new study results and when deciding where to go and receive care. We need quality and evidenced based care without perverse incentives.

Transparency Pledges

Dr. Marty Makary promoted the Transparency Pledge program with the publication of his book, **Unaccountable** in 2010. There are two pledges: one for the individual physician/health care provider and one for hospitals. These pledges reflect Dr. Makary's research findings as a quality assurance officer at Johns Hopkins Hospital in Baltimore, MD. So, the pledge signifies a commitment to quality patient care outcomes.

Transparency Pledge for Healthcare Providers

To increase transparency and trust with patients and community, I pledge to engage in the following best practices with my patients:

I pledge to disclose medical errors to patients as soon as I know about them

I pledge to disclose any money I receive from pharmaceutical or medical device company related to a patient's treatment options directly to the patient

I pledge to use internal hospital reporting systems to report hazards that I believe can harm patients

I pledge to openly and freely share a patient's medical record with the patient

I pledge to offer our patients a copy of their procedure video when video technology is used for medical care

I pledge to participate in the safety culture survey offered at my medical center

Transparency Pledge for Hospitals

To increase transparency and trust with our patients and community, our medical center's leadership pledges to engage in the following best practices:

We pledge to disclose medical errors to patients as soon as we know about them

We pledge to disclose all financial conflicts of interests to our patients

We pledge to make our patient outcomes available to the public through validated public reporting programs

We pledge to adopt open notes to streamline patient access to their health records

We pledge to offer our patients a copy of their procedure video when video technology is used for medical care

We pledge to adopt patient-centered care of hospitalized patients by encouraging a family member to stay with their loved one and by decreasing restrictions on family visitation hours

We pledge to measure hospital safety culture using validated methods

We pledge to participate in national quality improvement collaborative so that best practices can be studied and adopted

www.TransparentMillenium@gmail.com

Total Transparency Manifesto

Another physician, Dr. Leana Wen, has begun a Transparency Manifesto campaign on her website, www.whosmydoctor.com . Dr. Wen seeks to rebuild professionalism, prioritize patient values and respect human dignity in healthcare. I applaud her efforts to assist patients who feel vulnerable, powerless, and afraid when illness occurs to them or a loved one. Please visit her website and support her Total Transparency Manifesto if you agree.

We are patients and providers who believe that doctors need to be honest, transparent, and accountable.

When we go to the doctor, we are vulnerable and need to trust that our doctors have our best interests at heart.

Doctors have to tell each other at conferences if they are paid by drug companies or medical device companies; they should also tell their patients about these potential conflicts of interest. They need to be open with patients if their employers pay them more to do more, or to do less. These incentives directly affect patient care.

We believe that informed consent isn't complete without doctors' disclosure of how their financial incentives align with their treatment recommendations.

We also believe that patients have a right to know our doctors' views on healthcare issues such as preventive health, integrative medicine, shared decision-making, end-of-life care, and women's health. Such beliefs can have an important impact on the provider-patient relationship, and patients need ready access to this information to be empowered to choose the right doctor for us.

Those of us who are doctors, nurses, healthcare providers, and providers-in-training affirm through Who's My Doctor and this Total Transparency Manifesto that our patients' best interests are our best interests. We know that patients come to us at a time of vulnerability, so we will be vulnerable too. This is a partnership; we are in this together.

With this pledge, we are coming together as patients, doctors, and healthcare providers to rebuild our healthcare system into one that upholds professionalism, prioritizes patient values, and respects human dignity.

Performance Metrics

There is a famous business axiom that you can't improve it if you can't measure it.

Measurement and evaluation are two critical steps that improve our healthcare system. So, let's look at what we can measure in healthcare to determine quality care outcomes and patient satisfaction. Consumers can use public data on price, safety, quality indicators, and satisfaction scores to make informed decisions about the care they receive. As Dr. Makary reminds us, the best way to get a CEO's attention is to demand performance metrics **before you receive care** in his/her facility.

A recent article in the "Journal of Patient Safety," estimates that **440,000 consumers die from preventable medical errors in US hospitals**. This is now the **3rd leading cause of death** in the US behind cancer and heart disease. It eclipses deaths due to auto accidents and everything else. These deaths are not due to the reason for hospitalization such as an illness or injury, but rather hospital errors. These preventable errors include leaving sponges in surgical patients, medication dose errors or receiving the wrong medication, as well as hospital infections and falls or other injuries.

If I haven't already got your attention, listen to this. The cost of these grave errors is shifted to the consumer or taxpayer, and/or business paying for the care, the insurers. These hidden surcharges that Americans are paying for hospital errors have been calculated to be approximately

$500 million per year. A recent American Medical Association study found that employers paid $39,000 extra every time an employee suffered a surgical site infection. That's quite a perverse incentive for bad care!

Today, there are proven strategies for improving patient safety both in and out of the hospital. Those hospitals that follow safety guidelines show good results in reducing medical errors. So, informed health care consumers need to take charge of the hospital market place and insist on safety as a priority. **Consumers can let providers, hospitals, and medical device makers know they earn our business by delivering safe and quality care as evidenced by quality performance metrics.** We are not interested in paying for poor perfomers.

Here is a partial listing of some of these organizations at this time. In Chapter 9, you will learn more about this important consumer role in monitoring healthcare performance.

Compare Hospital Website: CMS

The Center for Medicare and Medicaid Services (CMS) website compares Medicare hospitals for the consumer based on two government programs to monitor hospital quality and safety. The first initiative the Hospital Readmissions Reduction Program began in October 2012. This program reduces payments to hospitals that treat Medicare patients and had excess readmissions for heart attack, heart failure, and pneumonia. Under this federal program, hospitals are financially penalized for such unnecessary and sometimes preventable readmissions.

In Fiscal Year 2014 a new federal program, "**Hospital Value Based Purchasing**" began. Hospital payments are based on performance in **three domains that reflect hospital quality:** the **clinical process of care domain; the patient experience of care domain**; and the **outcome domain**. The Total performance score (TPS) is derived from a 45% weight given to clinical process measurements, 30% patient experience data, and 25% weighted score for patient outcome measurements. So be sure to visit the www.Medicare.gov website and check out your hospital's **Total Performance Score.**

Leapfrog Group

The Leapfrog Group has become a national leader and advocate in hospital transparency. It is an independent not-for-profit organization founded in 2003 by the nation's leading employers and private healthcare experts. Their goal is to make "leaps" forward in hospital safety, quality and affordability in the US by promoting **transparency and value-based hospital incentives.**

The Leapfrog Group assigns each hospital a hospital safety score which grades hospitals on the extent of their errors. This score incorporates both process or structural measures and outcome measures. **Process measures** include **physician staffing levels, computerized physician data order entry, and various safe practice protocols.** **Outcome measures** include various clinical problems such as **air embolism, pressure sores, falls and trauma, surgical death rates, and post- operative rates for respiratory failure, pulmonary embolism, poor wound healing, and accidental puncture or laceration.**

Truven Health Analytics Rankings

Truven delivers unbiased information and **quantitative measures** like there trademarked, "100 Top Hospitals." These rankings seek to **improve both the cost and quality** of healthcare in your area. Each year, Truven conducts a study with a team of researchers that evaluates hospital performance using public data and the top 100 Hospitals'

National Balanced Scorecard. Public data sources include **Medicare cost reports, Medicare Provider Analysis and Review (MedPAR)** data, and **Centers for Medicare and Medicaid Services (CMS) Hospital Compare website core measures and patient satisfaction scores.**

The quantitative measures include excellence in clinical care, patient experience, operational efficiency, and financial stability. Annually, they name Everest Award winners and recognize hospitals with the highest one year performance and fastest long-term improvement over a period of five years. Last year, only 17 of the Top 100 Hospitals received the 2013 Everest Award. As we implement health care reform, it is important to monitor a hospital-wide culture of excellence from patient care experiences to housekeeping, and adopt evidence based hospital policies and procedures that assure patient safety and quality care outcomes.

Consumer Reports on HCAHPS Results

These hospital rankings are based on **patient safety scores** as well as **patient experience scores, patient outcomes,** and certain **hospital practices.** Consumer Reports rely on scientifically based data on patient experience collected from public sources. One example is the government survey, the **Hospital Consumer Assessment of Healthcare Providers and Systems (HCAHPS)** recently developed by **AHRQ.** These surveys come from patients with recent hospital stays. Patients assign a numeric score between zero and ten to recommend a hospital based on their recent experience. The parameters measured include:

Communication about discharge and medications

Doctor-patient and nurse-patient communication

Pain control

Timeliness of help you did or did not receive

Quietness of your hospital room at night

Cleanliness of your hospital room and bathroom

These publicly available patient satisfaction scores or HCAHPS now determine hospital reimbursements.

Consumer Reports Hospital Rankings

Consumer Reports hospital ranking system assigns a safety score on a **100 point scale** based on five categories: **avoiding infections, avoiding readmissions, explaining**

medications and discharge instructions, and using chest and abdominal scans appropriately. Complications score is worth 10 points and communication, infections, scanning and readmissions share the remaining 90 points. The rankings also look at **two hospital practices - appropriate use of scans** as well as **electronic medical records.** Scanning use is gleaned from billing date from CMS records that calculates the percent of CT scans of the abdomen and thorax that are performed twice. Such double scans are rarely necessary and evidence supports scanning with or without contrast dye, but not both. Unnecessary double scans expose patients to excess radiation and the potential adverse effects of the contrast dye.

Patient **outcome measures** look at **blood stream infections, surgical site infections, readmission** rates, and **eight serious complications**: bed sores, collapsed lungs, bloodstream infections, accidental punctures or cuts during surgery, post- surgery complications – post op infections, hip fractures, blood clots in the lungs or legs, and poor wound healing.

So there is a wealth of helpful information for consumers to view before they make an informed decision about where to go for their hospital care. These rankings also emphasize the importance of effective communication with patients and their families at the time of admission and discharge. This assures a good understanding what kind of care is needed and why, along with the common side effects of that care. We will discuss more about this in the next chapter.

U.S. News and World Reports Hospital Rankings

For years, consumers have been purchasing the annual *US News and World Reports* hospital rankings to shop for providers and facilities. Here is what I learned researching their methodology. These hospital rankings started in 1990 to **identify the best medical centers for the most difficult patients** – those whose unusual challenges like underlying conditions, procedure difficulty, or other medical issues – added to their risk. That is why these lists initially appeared as Best Hospitals. The focus of these lists has not changed.

The 2014 Executive Summary emphasizes that the rankings today still use measures of performance in structure, process and outcomes for 12 of the specialties. The remaining 4 specialities – **Opthamology, Psychiatry, Rehabilitation and Rheumatology – do not depend on objective data. Instead these hospitals are ranked solely by hospital reputation as determined by a physician survey.** Dr. Herzlinger warned us about the risk of only using industry wide data instead of independent sources of performance data.

In fact, the structural measures about hospital volume, technology, and other resources that define the hospital environment are derived from another biased industry source, the American Hospital Association's annual survey. *US News and World Reports* does state that they supplement these industry driven data sources with additional independent resources like the National Cancer Institute's list of designated cancer centers that meet specific criteria.

The process measures are determined by the hospital's reputation for developing and sustaining a system that delivers high quality care once again determined by a survey of board-certified physicians or providers. So, beware that this peer review process is subjective data not hard data from an independent source.

Finally, the *US News and World Reports* outcome performance measures rely on **risk adjusted mortality data from the Medicare Provider Analysis and Review (MedPar) database maintained by the Centers for Medicare and Medicaid Services (CMS).** Since the number of **elements of patient safety component** has increased, the 2014 rankings were revised to give more overall weight to these **objective data driven analytics**. This shift represents "improved reliability and accuracy of data-driven measures."

So, a word of caution to be careful and examine the source of the data you use when you compare hospitals and providers. Always look for hard data, objective measurements by independent groups versus subjective measurements like peer review studies and industry surveys.

Magnet Nursing Hospitals

Nurses provide care, prevent illness, and manage the health care delivery environment. This care coordination role has become increasingly important to patient safety. The Institute of Medicine Report in 2004 was the first to connect nursing practices with patient safety and quality of care. Certain characteristics of nursing organization and management as well as nurse staffing levels contribute to a safe care environment.

A 1983 nursing research study identified the **Magnet Characteristics of a Professional Practice Environment**. This list identified corporate cultures within health care organizations like hospitals which supported excellence in nursing and noticed a favorable impact on patient outcomes. By 1994 the American Nurses Association Credentialing Center started the Magnet Hospital Program. To date, only **225 organizations have achieved this designation.**

The Magnet Recognition Program recognizes health care organizations for **quality patient care, nursing excellence, and innovation in professional nursing practice**. Consumers can rely on this designation as the ultimate credential for high quality nursing. Please visit their website at www.nursecredentialing.org to find a Magnet Hospital near you.

Choosing Wisely Campaign

The National Physicians Alliance conceived and piloted a concept of a list of steps physicians in internal medicine, family medicine and pediatrics could implement in their practices to promote the most effective use of health care resources and improve quality of care. These lists were first published in the *Archives of Internal Medicine* These lists promote conversations between physicians and consumers to **choose care that is evidenced based, not duplicative of other tests and procedures, free from medical harm, and truly necessary.** In 2012 the Choosing Wisely Campaign began.

Consumer Reports is working with the Choosing Wisely Campaign to develop patient friendly materials to give to consumers. Consumers and physicians should use the recommendations as guidelines to determine an appropriate and personalized treatment plan. The March 2013 Consumer Reports issue recommended the following screening tests for most healthy consumers:

Cervical Cancer

Colon Cancer

Breast Cancer

It cautioned consumers to ask their primary care doctor to determine a personalized list of cancer screenings appropriate for them based on their personal, genetic, or family history risk factors.

Choosing Wisely Top 5 lists now represent specialty physician societies as well as the original primary care physician groups – internal medicine, family medicine, and pediatrics.

Please visit the website at www.choosingwisely.org/doctor-patientlists.org for these patient friendly resources. The lists include guidelines for the following common tests: allergy, colonoscopy, bone-density, echocardiograms, EKG, pap exams, spirometry, brain scans, and stress testing for chest pain. Imaging guidelines include heart, breast cancer tumor markers, headache, early prostate cancer, lower back pain, and ovarian cysts. Necessary treatment guidelines include migraine headaches, sinusitis, erection problems, blocked leg arteries, and heartburn/GERD. Other topics available include cancer care versus supportive care, chronic kidney disease hard choices, Immunoglobulin G (IgG) replacement therapy, and scheduling early delivery of your baby.

This group also publishes list of "**Five Things Physicians and Patients Should Question.**" Here are some of their lists:

American Academy of Family Physicians

Don't do imaging tests for low back pain within the first 6 weeks unless there is a red flag –severe neurological deficits or underlying condition like osteomyelitis

Don't routinely prescribe antibiotics for acute mild-to-moderate sinusitis unless symptoms last for 7 or more days, or worsen after initial clinical improvement

Don't use DEXA screening for osteoporosis in women less than 65 or men less than 70 with no risk factors

Don't order annual EKG or other cardiac screening for low-risk patients without symptoms

Don't perform Pap smears on women less than 21 or who have had a hysterectomy for a non-cancer disease

American Academy of Allergy, Asthma and Immunology

Don't perform unproven tests like IgG or IgE tests in allergy evaluations

Don't order sinus CT or indiscriminately prescribe antibiotics for uncomplicated acute symptoms

Don't routinely do diagnostic testing in patients with chronic urticarial (itching)

Don't recommend replacement immunoglobulin therapy for recurrent infections unless impaired antibody responses to vaccines are demonstrated

Don't diagnose or manage asthma without spirometry

American Gastroenterological Association

Treat GERD (acid reflux disease) by titrating the dose of long-term acid suppression therapy like Nexium and Pepsid to the lowest effective dose

Do not repeat colorectal cancer screening for 10 years after a high-quality colonoscopy is negative in average-risk individuals

Do not repeat colonoscopy for at least 5 years for patients with 1 or 2 small (less than 1cm) adenomatous polyps, without high-grade dysplasia, which were completely removed with a high-quality colonoscopy

Patients diagnosed with Barrett's esophagus with a second endoscopy with negative biopsy findings for dysplasia should have a follow-up exam in 3 years

Patients with functional abdominal pain syndrome, don't repeat CT scans unless there is a major change in clinical symptoms or findings

American Academy of Cardiology

Don't perform stress cardiac imaging or advanced non-invasive imaging in the initial evaluation of patients without cardiac symptoms unless high-risk markers are present

Don't perform annual stress cardiac imaging or advanced non-invasive imaging in routine follow-up in asymptomatic patients

Don't perform stress cardiac imaging or advanced non-invasive imaging as a pre-op assessment in patients scheduled for low-risk non-cardiac surgery

Don't perform echocardiography as routine follow-up for mild, asymptomatic native (not artificial) valve disease in adult patients with no change in signs or symptoms

Don't perform stenting of non-culprit lesions for percutaneous coronary intervention (PCI) for uncomplicated hemodynamically stable ST-segment elevation MI (STEMI)

American College of Physicians

Don't obtain screening exercise EKG testing in asymptomatic patients and at low risk for coronary heart disease

Don't get imaging studies in patients with non-specific low back pain

In the evaluation of simple syncope (fainting) with a normal neurological exam, don't obtain brain imaging studies (CT or MRI)

In patients with low pretest probability of venous thromboembolism (VTE), obtain a high high-sensitive D-dimer measurement initially not imaging studies

Don't obtain preoperative chest radiography in the absence of a clinical suspicion for intra thoracic pathology

Chapter 5 Health Challenge Goal: I challenge you to ask for a financial disclosure statement or pledge from your doctor or hospital before accepting a new treatment.

Chapter 6: Transparent Healthcare Navigation

A questioning man is half way to being wise.

Jonathan Swift

An investment in knowledge pays the best interest

Benjamin Franklin

Our present healthcare system performs poorly in terms of communication, coordination, and delivering healthy outcomes effectively and efficiently. As we learned in Chapter 2, data transparency can transform our healthcare system and make it more accountable. It also gives us the right to personalize our care with our values, care preferences, as well as genetic and family history data. This allows us to take charge of our own healthcare decisions. The last chapter has reminded us about the importance of quality, accurate, and current evidenced based information without undue financial strings. We need to insist on evidenced based best practices in care as the norm, not the exception. So, now is the time to do your homework before you seek care. Know what you want and need and ask for it.

In this chapter, we will discuss the need for data transparency, how to navigate modern healthcare successfully, and how to personalize your care to reflect your healthcare risks, preferences, and values to avoid unwanted care.

OPEN RECORDS

This was already discussed in Chapters 2 and 4 as a solution that works. Look for practices that provide you with data transparency with each visit. This might include:

A record of each visit printed at the conclusion of your visit listing your biometrics, clinical diagnosis for the visit, recommended treatment guidelines, and follow-up care timelines.

Copies of all test results in written format or on a disk with visual test results like a colonoscopy and MRI

An Open records policy usually means you can review your record to check for accuracy. My personal experience with an inadvertent medical record error convinced me that this is an important safeguard. When I went for my yearly physical several years ago, my doctor asked why I had an ER visit earlier in the year. My response was I had not visited an ER, but had called the after-hours MD to decide whether to take my child to the ER. So, I asked him to make a correction in my medical record and delete that misinformation. Yes, mistakes can and will happen and reviewing the record in a timely manner gives you the opportunity to make an immediate correction.

A June 10, 2014 article in the *Wall Street Journal* entitled, "Look in Your Medical Record, Odds are You'll Find a Mistake," by Laura Landro revealed a startling statistic, **errors can occur in 95% of medication lists in medical records. These errors could be outdated prescriptions, incorrect dosage or frequency.** Many large medical providers including Cleveland Clinic, Mayo Clinic, the Veterans Health Administration, Geisinger Health System, and Kaiser Permanente are giving **patients direct online access to their doctor's notes.** The purpose is to allow patients to correct or add to their records. This is a positive step towards the concept of "shared accountability" for effective care.

The most common errors include:

New prescription medicines aren't listed or old ones removed

An incorrect or outdated dosage of a prescription medicine

Duplicate prescriptions for brand name and generic medications

Over the counter (OTC) remedies aren't listed

Incomplete and missing information about medication allergies

Erroneous information about treatment outcome such as resolved, but it is still a problem

Updated information about lab results is missing

Details about patient symptoms are missing

Inaccuracies in diagnosis

Missing information or updates from another provider, such as a specialist. This is a positive and needed change in my opinion. My personal experience has given me two reasons to support this data transparency about prescription drugs in medical records. My elderly mother was given a medication she was allergic to during an ER visit because the hospital had not updated her medical record with the drug allergy that occurred in their ER during a prior visit!!

My husband had an abnormal test result that his own physician thought was a fluke. When I mentioned that this medication had a black box warning about this abnormal test result, I got his attention. He agreed with my suggestion to discontinue the medication for 30 days and repeat the lab test. Fortunately, the lab result returned to normal range. My husband's doctor's main question was "am I the prescribing MD?" He wasn't but, the medication was on my husband's medication list in his medical record with the practice group. We asked that his medical record reflect this drug reaction and a warning not to take this medication again.

Patients that have access to their own records are more likely to ask questions, identify errors or omissions, and give additional information that might affect the data in their records according to the National Operation Records Center (NORC) at the University of Chicago. This research organization is on contract with the National Coordinator for Health Information Technology. Patients in focus groups testing the open records approach commented that the **access to the medication list better prepared them for doctor visits and helped them be more proactive in managing their care.** Doctors are hoping to reduce malpractice liability by having more accurate medication information.

Another initiative called **"Open Notes"** is currently allowing 168,000 patients to view their doctor's notes online through a secure patient portal. Patients will be encouraged to add their own notes including family caregiver notes asking for corrections for patients too ill to make their own comments. Patients in the study are checking OpenNotes to review what was said during and after the appointment. **Patients are noticing the results of abnormal test results sometimes before their provider!** Now that is true patient engagement at its best!!

WHERE IS YOUR MEDICAL HOME?

The ACA introduced the concept of a Medical Home which is based on studies of what creates a highly performing healthcare system. The Agency for Healthcare Research and Quality (AHRQ) defines the medical home as a model organization of primary care that delivers the core functions of primary health care. These five functions can be used as a **yardstick for selecting a primary care practice.**

Comprehensive Care is provided by a team of care providers which meets the physical and mental needs of its members. This care encompasses prevention and wellness, as well as, acute and chronic care.

Patient-centered or care of the whole person is based on a partnership with patients respecting their **unique needs, culture, values, and preferences**. It actively **supports patient learning to manage and organize their own level of care in a care plan they choose.** The team also informs family members if the patient desires.

Coordinated care across the health care system including **specialty care, hospitals, home health care, and community services**. This coordination is critical during transitions in care like home to hospital, ER to hospital, or hospital to rehab or nursing home. Clear and open communication is fostered between patients, the medical home, and the delivery system.

Accessible services with **shorter wait times for urgent needs, enhanced in-person visits, 24/7 telephone or electronic access to care team members, and timely response to patient preference for desired level of access** are delivered by the medical home care team.

Quality and safety commitment is demonstrated by using **evidenced-based medicine** and clinical decision tools to **support shared decision making with patients**.

Measuring performance, responding to patient satisfaction comments, practicing population health management, and sharing quality and safety data publicly are all part of this model.

Therefore, a healthcare team approach with better communication methods, better response time, and documentation of health changes would clearly improve our present healthcare system performance and accountability to the consumer. If you are wondering where to **find a certified patient centered medical home (PCMH) practice near you**, here is a website to check: www.ncqa.org. The National Committee for Quality Assurance is a private non-profit organization dedicated to improving health care quality. Their direct approach motto is: measure, analyze, improve, and repeat! The NCQA seal is a widely recognized symbol of quality that revolves around quality standards and performance measures. Their seal of approval for health plans has to meet a rigorous set of over 60 standards and must report their performance in more than 40 areas to earn their seal of approval.

My care is delivered in a medial home certified practice. At the conclusion of each health visit, I receive a written summary of my visit. This summary includes my biometric measurements, clinical diagnosis, treatment recommendations, and any follow-up care needed as well as contact information for any referrals made. It gives me the opportunity to correct any mistakes in my record immediately after my visit. In fact, I have included this as one of the Healthcare-Equalizer Consumer Bill of Rights in Chapter 7!

SELECTING YOUR PCP

As we move towards a prevention model of health care, it is paramount that you have a primary care physician. This person is the hub of your care, coordinating reports from various specialists as well as the keeper of your personal, family medical histories, and genetic data. This person is in the best position to evaluate new symptoms that occur and can evaluate them against the backdrop of your chronic conditions, significant family medical history, and test results.

An old adage for picking a general doctor was to pick someone whose practice was close to your home, experienced, board certified in internal or family medicine, and had a part time teaching position with a university medical school. This prescription assumed the practitioner was competent, experienced, and interested in keeping current with changes in medical practices. These criteria are still vital, but today there are additional criteria for the cost conscious insured consumer.

Today, you need to **check whether your insurance has a network of preferred providers whose visits are covered completely. Usually out of network providers usually incur a larger copay and less coverage, usually about 80% coverage after a deductible has been applied**. So, it pays to study your health plan carefully before deciding who your primary care practitioner will be. **This concern is especially important when you visit an ER or enter a hospital. You need to verify that individual physician providers are part of your network, not just the hospital ER.**

An additional concern is whether the primary care practice has the features you desire. This list may include evening and Saturday hours, a doctor call-in time, a nurses' line, additional services onsite such as blood drawing, x-ray, physical therapy, etc. It is also a good idea to check the practice website for various business fees such as cancelled appointments, fees for form completions for school and employer physicals, and facility fees. The latter has become a practice among large urban medical centers and not usually found in community practices in the suburbs.

YOUR PHYSICAL EXAM VISIT

An initial interview with a new healthcare provider is an opportunity for you to find one that supports your philosophy of care and values about healthcare. Do you favor behavioral changes such as nutrition, exercise, and other lifestyle habits, over simply medication based treatments? Do you want to evaluate the pre-treatment costs before deciding what type of care? Do you want information on side effects and possible complications from a proposed treatment or screening procedure before you make your decision? Are they willing to develop personalized screening recommendations based on your risk factors? Are they willing to create a chronic disease action plan with you?

A prevention model of health care emphasizes a physical exam every year or two to evaluate your health and health risks. As we discussed in Chapter 4, this is the time to discuss your written RNA and Chronic Disease Action Plans. This visit should also discuss any new genetic or family history information as well as measure your current biometrics. Your RNA can be examined to determine whether those habits reduce your controllable risk factors. Some target biometrics can be set as target goals for the next checkup.

It is also wise to check your current immunization recommendations and decide whether any new vaccines are appropriate for you given your age and health risks. This visit should discuss any new symptoms or changes in your body or mental health issues that you have noticed. So, be prepared and bring your list of questions with you. Ask your provider for 5 minutes of the exam visit to discuss your written questions. Lastly, a checkup should include a schedule for regular dental and eye exams and a discussion of safety features to follow like seatbelts, bike helmets, and smoke alarms.

MEDICATIONS 101

A 2013 CDC report notes that almost 48% of Americans take at least one prescription drug and that 10% of those taking prescription drugs take 5 or more! The CDC attributes three factors with this doubling of our prescription drug national expenditure from 5.6% in 1990 to 9.7% by 2010:

New and innovative drug therapies available for infections and chronic diseases

Expansion in drug coverage in public and private insurance plans

Exponential growth of pharmaceutical marketing directly to consumers by 300%

Along with our $280 billion national expenditure on drugs in 2013, we are now facing issues related to the abuse of prescription drugs including:

Overuse of antibiotics for viral infections has led to the development of antibiotic resistant infections

Opoid analgesic pain relief abuse increased 300% between 1999 and 2010 and deaths due to opoids also increased 300% in the same time period

85% of people with mental health conditions are now treated with drugs with powerful side effects

Medication side effects can include acid reflux, headache, nausea, bowel changes, neurologic symptoms like muscle weakness and nerve pain, ringing in the ears, dizziness, sleepiness and anxiety. Medications should be dosed according to your weight. So, if you are a small lightweight adult like me, be sure to notify your provider that you want an appropriate dose. Side effects are more common at higher dosages. Also, elderly patients often lose weight due to poor eating habits or lack of appetite. Be sure to revisit dosages with their primary care provider with each visit.

Be sure to check the information your pharmacy provides with each prescription drug. Pay special attention to any drug contraindications and serious side effects. A black box warning on the label usually lists serious and sometimes rare side effects that can be life threatening.

Remember my experience with my husband's abnormal blood test result! Ask your doctor to give you drugs that you can take during the work day. You don't want to take prescription drugs that cause dizziness, sleepiness, and poor reflexes if you are working with equipment or have job responsibilities requiring focus and attention for critical decisions. Also, ask your doctor or pharmacist how long you should take the medication. Some drug side effects become more common with continued drug use. Be sure to ask about other non-drug treatment options in case the medication doesn't help you or the drug has undesirable side effects.

Polypharmacy – Taking Multiple Drugs

Be sure to ask your doctor and pharmacist to revisit the individual dose of each drug. Also, ask your pharmacist about the best time of day to take the drug for maximum effectiveness. You may be able to get relief at lower doses when taken appropriately. Be sure to heed the cautions on many pain reliever drugs and mental health drugs prohibiting use with alcohol.

A Johns Hopkins Health Alert on the dangers of polypharmacy cautions consumers that older people tend totake more medications, metabolize drugs less efficiently, and are more likely to experience drug-drug interactions. This is when one medication affects the way another medication works or makes the effect of that medication more pronounced.

Some symptoms that could indicate your drugs aren't mixing well with you include a rash, fever, diarrhea, mild breathing difficulty, and a rapid or slow heartbeat. More serious drug reactions include seizures and anaphylactic shock which can be fatal. Anaphylactic shock usually accompanies drug allergic reactions and cause life threatening breathing problems, heartbeat irregularities, and systemic body rashes. I have had these scary reactions and always remember to list my known drug allergies with each provider or healthcare facility I visit.

Even mild symptoms like drowsiness and dizziness can increase the likelihood of patient injury or harm from a fracture or fall. These events can lead to a cycle of disability and declining health. In fact, a recent study looked at the aftereffects for patients that had experienced medical errors, such as medication errors, and found their mortality rate often increased.

If the drug is the culprit for your new symptom, check with your provider about other ways to tackle the symptom besides a drug. You might be surprised at the options today! Some alternative treatments can be very effective for controlling anxiety, lower back pain, chronic pain, and mild depression. Consumers don't need to listen to TV commercials to find drugs or medical devices to take for their chronic condition.

Consult your healthcare provider and do your own research on the USPHS website, our prevention bible, where you can find letter graded scientific evidence for the best treatments of various chronic conditions.

OTC Cold Medication Dangers

A recent article exposed some of the hidden dangers in common cold remedies. Tylenol or acetaminophen has a maximum safe daily dose of 3000-4000mg. Overdoses can lead to toxicity and sometimes severe liver damage. Stay away from alcohol is you are taking Tylenol and use the lowest dose that gives relief. Read the label carefully and make sure you are aware of all medications you may be taking that contain Tylenol.

Advil or ibuprofen is a non-steroidal anti-inflammatory drug or (NSAID) that is quite effective for body aches, headaches, and fever. It can cause severe allergic reactions as well as peptic ulcers and kidney damage with chronic use. It may increase the chance for a heart attack or stroke if you have high blood pressure, heart disease, are a smoker or have diabetes.

Decongestants like Triaminic and Dimetapp can relieve nasal congestion by constricting blood vessels in the nose.

This can also cause blood pressure to rise and interfere with the effectiveness of prescription drugs to control blood pressure. Decongestant nasal sprays like Afrin and Neo-Synephrine cause fewer side effects, but be careful about rebound congestion if you use them for more than 3 days.

Antihistamines like Benadryl and Chlor-Trimeton block histamine and relieve runny and itchy noses. These older antihistamines cause drowsiness, impair coordination, and slow reaction times which increase the risk of falls in older people. Don't use these shorter acting antihistamines if you have glaucoma, an enlarged prostate, high blood pressure, or heart disease. Longer acting newer antihistamines like Claritin, Zyrtec, and Allegra taken once a day don't cause drowsiness.

Many OTC cold remedies contain combinations of drugs like antihistamines with decongestants and can cause irregular heartbeats, high blood pressure, and tremors.

Finally, consider using a single ingredient medication to control the most bothersome symptom.

Self-Care and Monitoring

You live with your body 24/7 so you are the best judge of any change in its normal behavior. So promise to commit yourself to finding the root cause of new symptoms instead of just treating a new symptom. Some problems can be cured once you treat the root cause.

New Symptoms

As an experienced nurse, I have listened to countless patients with new symptoms. New symptoms fall into 3 major categories in my mind: emergency, urgent, and wait and see.

Emergency Symptoms

Severe breathing difficulties

Loss of consciousness

Injuries with significant blood loss and/or broken bones

Sudden changes in cognition – **FAST** approach to stroke detection

Facial drooping

Arm weakness and/or numbness

Speech problems

Time to call 911

Severe headache with dizziness

Sudden loss of vision or hearing

Allergic reactions to drugs, animal or insect bites, foods, or chemicals are called anaphylaxis. These symptoms may include breathing difficulties, throat constriction, fainting, and loss of consciousness. Some life threatening reactions need prompt attention. Use your emergency medications like an Epi pen or Benadryl pill and then call your doctor's office or visit your closest emergency room.

Urgent Symptoms

These are conditions that can easily be treated in an urgent care setting:

Common infections – eye, sinus, throat, respiratory, ear, vaginal and urinary tract

Mild breathing changes

Coughing that disrupts your sleep

Allergy symptoms – nasal stuffiness, swollen itchy eyes and ears, nasal drip

Acid reflux and GI issues that disrupt sleep and eating habits

Muscle and bone injuries

Call your membership services phone number on your insurance card to find out which urgent care clinics are in-network and what the copay will be. Most urgent care clinics have a list of standard fees for different services that you can inspect prior to accepting care. Beware of urgent care centers that don't list their prices because they may be much higher than other centers.

Wait and See Symptoms

These are symptoms that you can manage at home and observe for serious changes that warrant a future provider visit. Measuring and evaluating new symptoms is imperative before seeking care from your provider. Here are some common wait and see symptoms:

Cold symptoms – nasal congestion, coughing, itchy throat

Minor injuries with bruising and pain following trauma

Overuse injuries with pain and sometimes weakness and tingling

GI upsets with belching, constipation, nausea, and diarrhea

Minor Injuries

With recent injuries, your best first response is RICE.

R = rest the injured body part for at least 30 minutes and assess

I = Ice for 24-48 hours. This controls inflammation which causes pain and also prevents complications from soft tissue injuries (muscles, tendons, ligaments). The proper instructions for icing include ice the area for 15 minutes every hour as needed. The longer you keep up this regimen, the more it will suppress the inflammation and swelling which greatly reduces your pain.

C = Compression. This involves wrapping the affected area to control swelling.

E = Elevation. The usual rule of thumb is to elevate the body part above the level of the heart for at least 30 minutes initially at the time of injury. This again suppresses inflammation and encourages circulation to the injured area.

Inflammation is the body's natural response to trauma. When you control inflammation quickly, the pain level is reduced and you often achieve a better range of motion sooner in the affected area. The RICE method is very effective, but often underused by patients. Another suggestion is to take an anti-inflammatory cream or pill that your doctor recommends for you. This regimen can add to the RICE treatment success in the first critical 24-48 hours after the injury.

My personal experience with the RICE formula has been quite successful. I have had two recent injuries, a tumble off a footstool hanging draperies and a collision with a bicyclist in Berlin after stepping off a curb. Both of these injuries caused intense pain and weakness initially, but a prompt RICE response and anti-inflammatory medication in the critical 24-48 hours reduced my pain level and dramatically reduced the amount of swelling and injury. Both of these injuries were fortunately smooth muscle and not broken bones. Initially, I was caught off guard by the intensity of the pain, but my deep breathing exercises calmed me so I could make smart decisions.

Practice the 4-7-8 deep breathing immediately to calm yourself

Ice the area 15 mins hourly for the next 24-48 hours until the swelling is gone

Elevate the injured area above the heart

Stay off the limb for the first 24 hours

Avoid weight bearing activities involving the area until pain is gone

Use an anti-inflammatory cream or drug your doctor recommends for you and follow the directions carefully

Resting injured body parts is invaluable for a complete recovery and achieving maximum range of motion in the affected part. Next, evaluate whether you have a broken bone by measuring the amount of swelling, pain, and inability to bear weight on the body area after this critical 24-48 hours. Always consult with your doctor's office when pain and swelling increase after this critical period.

Chronic Symptom Management

Headaches, gastrointestinal or GI symptoms like indigestion, diarrhea and vomiting, and minor aches and pains are part of our stressful lives. Lack of sleep, poor dietary practices, and lack of regular exercise can cause periodic symptoms like these as well as overuse injuries at work and home. For instance a lot of GERD symptoms could be relieved by not eating late at night. In fact, you should stop eating 2-3 hours before bedtime. So, ask yourself what might be the root cause for this new symptom and then treat that possible cause. If the symptoms worsen after a few days, consider contacting your healthcare provider to rule out more serious causes of the symptoms.

Some chronic diseases like diabetes, asthma, and high blood pressure can be easily monitored by the patient using a glucose meter, peak flow meter, or blood pressure gauge to measure changes in your biometrics. Design a chronic disease action plan that you read about in Chapter 4 and evaluate your measurement against the stoplight zones. You and your doctor can decide in advance how you should respond to yellow and red zone measurements of your target biometric. Self-monitoring like this can prevent serious complications and hospitalizations.

TRANSITION POINTS IN CARE

This is the new buzzword in healthcare administration. Care transitions have to be carefully managed to assure that the handoff in care is successful in communicating changes in the patient's care to the next provider. This process is rarely seamless and can be uncoordinated. This can result in delays in care, medical errors, and poor health outcomes that can harm patients. So, let's discuss some healthcare consumer skills to take charge of these transition points in care.

Monitor any Transfer of Care

Occasionally, consumers need care from a different facility or become dissatisfied with their care in a hospital or facility and desire to transfer to another facility. This situation usually has to be handled between physicians. Specifically, the sending physician initiates contact with the desired facility and requests a transfer of care. The receiving hospital decides whether they can or will accept the patient. Sometimes, patients are accepted for an outpatient evaluation versus an inpatient hospitalization.

In these circumstances, be sure to check whether your insurance plan will cover the cost of transport for a family request. Also, verify coverage for hospitalization coverage at this desired facility. Every transfer point in care demands careful exchange of important patient information. Just because a family member has transferred from another facility, do not assume that their advance directives and list of allergies and medications arrived with them. I have personally experienced the lack of these medical record documents missing from my mother's records when she was sent to an ER from her assisted living and dementia facilities. Family members must always keep a copy of these documents with them. Your car glove box is one safe storage place that is immediately available to you in an emergency. Hospitals can only respect them if they are aware of them. These documents represent your loved one's autonomy in directing their care. You will learn more about this topic in Chapter 7.

Drug allergies and other care contraindications are also vital and imperative to be transmitted to new temporary or permanent healthcare providers. These **care contraindications** may include:

Drug and latex allergies and chemical sensitivities

No blood pressure measurement in specific arm

Medical devices installed (spinal stimulators, defibrillator or pacemaker)

Religious preferences such as Jehovah Witness refusal for blood transfusions

Any mental health concerns or cognition deficits like autism, retardation, or dementia

These care transition points are the best time to arrange a meeting between the patient and a family member with the new healthcare team.

Admission Care Plan Meeting

The goal of this meeting should be the transfer of all important patient documents such as such as immunization record, current and accurate medication list with correct dosage and frequency, any DNR – do not resuscitate order - and of course any living directives.

The agenda is to discuss the plan of care and services that the patient is expected to receive. This list may include tests and procedures in addition to new drugs. Be sure to identify the family member who has the medical power of attorney or is the healthcare representative for the patient. This advocate should always be present during these care planning sessions to reduce errors and misunderstandings.

Patients always have the right to refuse or amend care ordered for them by their provider. When the new care setting is a hospital, a new doctor called the hospitalist, usually supervises the patient's care and writes new orders. Nursing units usually assign a registered nurse to each patient each day to manage their care plan. Introduce yourself to this caregiver and speak directly with the primary nurse with any daily questions or suggestions. You are responsible for clear and open communication with the healthcare team to personalize your own care or that of a loved one.

Patients also have the right to refuse to board in an ER when they are waiting for a bed in another facility. Ask lots of questions and exercise your rights to get the care you want and need. Some ERs have senior areas and some hospitals have palliative care floors so ask for these special services. Today, it also makes sense to call your member services phone number on your insurance card when you elect to change your care facility. Ask about expected charges and the network status of providers and facilities. This is valuable information that may affect your decision.

Discharge Care Plan Meeting

This meeting should be requested by the patient and their family at least 24 hours prior to discharge, if possible. It should involve the follow written information:

Name of attending physician in hospital or facility and phone number

Name of follow-up physician and contact information

Summary of care received during this ER visit or hospitalization

Support services ordered and their contact information for follow-up. This may include visiting nurse services, respiratory care equipment, physical or occupational therapy visits, etc.

Written patient education materials for wound care, nutrition changes, sleep recommendations or biometric measurements to monitor

Evaluation survey for patient and family to complete about recent care experience

Verification for desired pharmacy contact information and any changed insurance information

In healthcare, we learned that smooth transitions in care don't just happen. They occur because they are well planned, organized, and clearly communicated. **Consumers need to initiate these meetings at a care transition point to assure safe, quality, and personalized appropriate care.**

END-OF-LFE CARE

Palliative and Hospice Care

The Hospice movement is both ancient and modern according to joint authors, Maggie Callanan and Patricia Kelley, of **Final Gifts,** a wonderful book to understand death and dying. In Medieval times, weary and sometimes dying travelers needed a place of comfort with food, shelter and help. Europe was filled with hospices along the routes to the Holy Land. In the early 1800s, the Irish Sisters of Charity began hospices in Ireland and England. In 1960, a physician working in the St. Joseph's Hospice in London, Dr. Cicely Saunders, began the work of our modern day hospice movement.

Dr. Saunders proposed a new way to care for the dying and her first hospice, St. Christopher's, began in London in 1967. Her approach combined loving, compassionate care with medical palliative interventions that relieved symptoms instead of curative care. She told her patients, "You matter because you are. You matter until the last moment of your life, and we will do all we can not only to help you die peacefully, but also to live until you die." At the same time, Dr. Kubler Ross, a US psychiatrist, began writing about changing attitudes toward death and dying so that the hospice movement might flourish here. Her classic book, **On Death and Dying,** was mandatory reading for my nursing baccalaureate program. Dr. Ross noted that the dying were often isolated from other patients and heavily sedated for their pain and not included in decisions about procedures imposed on them. Dr. Ross proposed a new way to treat the death and dying patient with compassionate care, dignity, and patient centered services to meet their wishes.

The American Hospice Foundation provides the consumer with helpful information about end of life care. Here are some of the facts on their website:

90% of us die from long, slow illnesses instead of a sudden death

70% of Americans want to die at home, but only 25% actually do

Most hospice patients die at home surrounded by loved ones. Hospice care is a model for quality and compassionate care at the end of life using a team approach with expertise in medical care, pain management, and emotional and spiritual support expressly tailored to the needs of the patient and family. Once the World Health

Organization defined palliative care in 1990, it extended the principles of hospice care to a broader population of people who could benefit from such care earlier in their disease.

Hospice care addresses the physical, emotional, social, and spiritual pain to achieve the best possible quality of life for patient's wishes. These emotional and spiritual support resources are extended to the family and loved ones. Generally, the care is provided in the patient's home or a home like setting operated by a hospice program. Medicare, private and commercial insurance, and Medicaid in most states cover hospice care for patients who meet the medical criteria.

The patient or family starts the dialogue with the patient's physician. The physician completes paperwork that is submitted to hospice to consider a patient for its services. The assessment home or facility visit is conducted by a registered hospice nurse. Next, a meeting is arranged and conducted by the hospice team with the family and/or facility caregivers. The hospice team usually includes a registered nurse, a social worker, and a pastoral support person. The hospice team decides on the type and frequency of their services for each patient. The visits might be weekly by a hospice nurse to assess the patient and/or a specially trained volunteer to comfort and support the dying patient with dignity and compassion.

Many people mistakenly think that hospice care means the end to curative care. Choosing hospice care means stopping attempts to cure life-limiting illness like cancer (or whatever your doctor indicated is your terminal disease) in favor of comfort care and relief from symptoms. You can still receive curative care for other non-life limiting illnesses. Care is initially approved for a two 90-day periods of time. After 180 days, the doctor may recertify the patient for an indefinite number of additional 60 day periods of hospice care as long as the patient remains medically eligible.

Recent articles in the Washington Post and New York Times have warned consumers to comparison shop for their hospice care. Presently, there is no hospice compare tool for public data. However, the ACA requires such public reporting. Within the next two to four years, the Centers for Medicare and Medicaid (CMM) will publish such a tool.

Here are some tips to finding quality hospice care in your area:

Ask for the results of the hospice's own patient satisfaction survey

Find out how long they have been in business

Ask about staff response times in the evenings and on weekends

Ask about their policy for continuous care. This care is given when the patient is actively dying or their last hours of life. Some hospices choose not to provide continuous care especially in some states. So be sure to ask.

Do they have an inpatient facility if symptoms become complicated? Do they have the ability to manage the patient outside of the home?

Who does the respite visits and how often are they? These visits are the weekly or daily visits that the hospice team has ordered for the patient.

Ask your provider about the reputation of the hospice you are considering

How Not To Die

An April 2014 Atlantic Magazine article, "How Not to Die," by Jonathan Rauch featured an innovative video program by a husband and wife medical team from Harvard. Dr. Angelo Volandes and Dr. Angela Delight-Davis started a controversial conversation in the medical community. Their message to doctors was be honest and transparent about the efficacy of late disease interventions and the patient's quality of life. They also confronted the "unwanted care" that often accompanies hospital deaths.

Videos present a new manner of presenting difficult information in a context that is informative without being emotional. These short 6-7 minute videos explain in visual detail what the terms CPR, feeding tube, and mechanical ventilation or a respirator actually mean. It also presents evidence about their effectiveness in prolonging life and how the patient experiences it. Doctors Volandes and Davis found that after viewing these informative videos, most family members choose comfort care over aggressive and limited care. Several clinical trials have shown the effectiveness of their videos in assisting patients and their families as well as the medical teams with these difficult decisions.

These brave medical reformers exposed the huge problem we have in American medicine with unwanted care. Dr Atul Gawande in his new book, **Being Mortal,** also challenged the old-fashioned medical approach to treat anything that might be treatable, at any stage of life – even near the end, when there is little hope of cure. Patients often feel powerless and frustrated with these decisions about very, very sick loved ones. We can take charge of these decisions by making them in advance with an advance directive. Consumers can change the death experience in hospitals for their loved ones by having the conversation early with the medical team.

My siblings and I were able to give both of our parents a hospice death they chose surrounded by family. Our dad died at 71 from metastatic colon cancer. He chose to enroll in hospice about a month before this death. He invited my older sister and I to attend his hospice orientation because we had encouraged him to consider this option. My Mom's increasing dementia symptoms at age 86 prompted me to dialogue with her about her final wishes before she became cognitively unable to make her own decision. She confided to me that she wanted the same hospice death as our Dad. I made a promise to her that we would respect her final wishes. So, we sat down and wrote a living directive using her words and had it signed by her primary care physician.

My Mom's admission to Hospice services didn't occur until several years later at age 89 when she had a life threatening gastrointestinal bleed. This medical event convinced her dementia facility MD to finally approve hospice for her despite my pleas to begin it sooner. She enjoyed three months of hospice services which included a more supportive wheelchair, a hospital type bed, and regular volunteer and hospice nurse visits. One of her volunteers played the harp which calmed her and brought her much joy.

When her final GI bleed occurred, the advanced planning made the final event progress smoothly and with less stress. The medications were on board in her dementia facility and the hospice nurse was a phone call away and directed the administration of medications by the dementia facility nurses. My family also had the opportunity to discuss comfort measures directly with the hospice staff during this time. Mom had the dignified, loving, and peaceful death she yearned to receive with her family at her bedside. It was an honor and privilege to witness the gift of a peaceful hospice death she desired and we had promised.

I want other families to know about this option. Hospice care is covered by Medicare and all insurances. **Start the dialogue today with you or your loved one's doctor, so they know your wishes. Visit www.fivewishes.org**

Advanced Care Directives

Each state also has a geriatrics or senior citizen services department. Here you can usually download the applicable state mandatory forms to document your end-of-life wishes. Be sure to give your family members, your primary physician, and your care facility a copy of this. Some people find in helpful to keep a copy in the car glove compartment if a loved one is terminally ill. A sudden trip to the emergency room doesn't have to mean you forgot the advanced care directive.

In Chapter 7, you will learn more about these living will directive forms and the importance of making sure they are respected and available to share with your provider in any setting.

TRAVEL SAFE: BE PREPARED

It is your responsibility to contact your insurer to find out what kind of coverage you have when outside your geographic area of coverage. Some insurance plans feature a suitcase logo for plans that are portable outside your state. Other plans operate on a reimbursement mode for out of the state or out of the country care. Some major insurers have a worldwide service level that allows you to get reimbursed for necessary care while abroad. Keep your receipts if you expect reimbursement.

Travel clinics can offer many services for certain vaccinations required for entry into certain countries. The CDC and State Department maintain websites with information for travelers about recommended or mandatory vaccinations and/or preventive medications. Travel Guard provides insurance plans for each trip and protection for medical transport services that might be needed. The World Health Organization (WHO) has a Travel and Health Guide which provides information on the health risks associated with each country and what you can do to prepare.

Frequent travel can wreak havoc with your health. Business travelers often experience jet lag, sleep disorders, increased alcohol and fast food intake, and long periods of sedentary living. Airplane travel gives the body a dehydrating experience. So, be sure to stay hydrated with water and avoid coffee and alcohol which can be dehydrating. These travel risk factors also raise blood pressure and increase the risk of obesity, so take your RNA plan with you on your next trip!

A potential life threatening risk for long-distance air travelers is a blood clot. Some risk factors for developing a blood clot are a family history of DVT (deep vein thrombosis), birth control pills, recent surgery and travel. Dehydration and cramped quarters in modern airplanes are partially to blame. The best prevention is stretching your leg and calf muscles every one to two hours. If getting up is difficult, do seated calf exercises such as flexing your toes up and down to encourage better circulation.

People with a higher risk for blood clots may consider wearing a compression stocking or sock that keeps blood from pooling in your legs. Be sure to discuss this with your health provider. Please pay close attention to any new symptoms since early and prompt actions can be lifesaving. Muscle soreness, redness, swelling, and pain in one leg should be watched closely and sometimes is treated with blood thinners. Be sure to discuss all the options for these drugs with your provider and find the best fit for you.

Another health concern is an airborne pathogen in the airplane. This can include the flu virus, tuberculosis bacterium, the antibiotic resistant superbug MRSA, and E. coli as well as Ebola virus, SARS (severe acute respiratory syndrome),and MERS (Middle East Respiratory Syndrome) virus. Two travel smart health behaviors recommended by microbiologist James Barbaree and his team at Auburn University include:

Use a hand sanitizer gel with 60% alcohol before you eat or drink and after using the airplane bathroom.

You can blow away airborne microbes by using the plane's recycled air. Set the vent above your head on the low or medium setting to create a current to knock harmful pathogens away.

Pack a medical kit that includes extra doses of regular medications you take, antibiotics, sterile bandages, wraps and an anti-inflammatory medication that works for you. Some travel experts recommend carrying a letter from your physician if you carry any medical equipment that could be ruined by airport scanners.

Chapter 6 Health Challenge Goal: I challenge you to find a medical home practice for your PCP.

Chapter 7: Your Healthcare Rights

Do not resent growing old. Many are denied the privilege

> Irish Proverb

Everyone has to contribute to the common good. With rights comes responsibility to our communities. When we're connected to others, we become better people.

> Randy Pasch, The Last Lecture

Then, join in the fight that will give you the right to be free!

"Do You Hear the People Sing," *Les Miserables*

PRIVACY

Healthcare privacy is a significant concern to most consumers. In this age of electronic record sharing, we must be careful about protecting the access to our personal medical information or PMI. Be sure to check with your provider's office about the choice to opt out of sharing your medical record information with other groups. There is usually a form you have to fill out limiting this sharing to what is medically necessary and also includes a provision that you will be notified about additional sharing that the practice initiates.

Age Related Privacy: College aged students (over 18) are allowed to have protected medical information privacy. So, as their parents, you are not allowed access to their medical information unless they notify the provider that you can access. Even though you may be paying for their healthcare plan, by law, the privacy of their medical information is protected.

HIPPA AND YOUR MEDICAL RECORD

The Health Insurance Portability and Protection Act (HIPPA) gave birth to the privacy concerns of your personal health information (PHI) and gave health providers the responsibility for protecting the privacy of that information with every exchange of information they create. Today, with the advent of electronic medical records, we now face a need to own and protect our medical data and information. This is privileged information about us. We need to see it and protect it and have access to it as much as we desire. Our non-transparent healthcare system has treated such information access as a secondary or reactive process in my opinion. Instead of us directing transfer of our PHI, we must rely on forms that providers issue for us to transfer our medical information.

What if we were to actually direct the transmission of our PHI and have to approve who we allowed to view and use our PHI? Consumers need to carefully monitor and sometimes choose to opt out of this sharing to assure we are in the driver's seat on this important topic. In the future, the concept of a health vault to store your PHI will become more popular and necessary. This cloud parking spot for your privileged health information will be necessary as electronic medical records become established as the norm.

MEDICAL POWER OF ATTORNEY

A medical power of attorney form can be filed in advance to appoint someone to act on your behalf should you become disabled or are unable to make your own medical decisions. This form usually needs to be notarized. Be sure your provider and any treatment facility keeps a copy in your medical record.

The person with the medical power of attorney should also keep a copy of this powerful document handy and available at a moment's notice. Accidents and changes in medical conditions can be unpredictable.

HEALTHCARE REPRESENTATIVE WITH YOUR INSURER

Individuals can assign a family member or friend to this role by filing a form with their insurance provider. The form usually has to be notarized and submitted to the insurer and can also be sent to the provider(s) to document who to contact about any aspect of the person's covered services under their health plan. I used this arrangement for my Mom as she became more confused and less able to conduct her health insurance affairs. My older sister, a CPA, was appointed by my Mom as her official power of attorney. My health insurance representative role merely made me the first point of contact about health bills and covered services with her health plan. Since I interact daily with the healthcare system, it was an easier task for me to perform. My sister and I were a great team and were able to resolve multiple incorrect bills and care disputes for our Mom. It also made it easier for caregivers to communicate directly with us instead of multiple family members.

Contact your insurance customer service center to get a copy of the appropriate form to complete which initiates this role you assume for your loved one. This healthcare representative can act on your behalf with respect to:

Making decisions about your health benefits

Requesting and/or disclosing your private health information

Exercising all of the rights you have under your health benefit plan

This power can be designated by the health care plan member directly when they sign the form in the presence of a Notary Public. A personal representative can also be legally appointed such as a medical-power-of-attorney and those forms can be submitted with this form as well.

ADVANCE OR END-OF-LIFE DIRECTIVES

Only 25% of consumers actually have end-of-life directives on file with their primary provider. The purpose of these notarized directives is to be your voice when these decisions need to made for you. These forms are readily available online at www.fivewishesfoundtion.org and your state's office of geriatrics and healthcare affairs. The form can be completed as I did with your loved one's actual words to indicate their final wishes.

Implementing these clear directives can be problematic. You need to keep a copy of this important form with you or on file during emergency room visits or at the time of hospitalization. A good rule of thumb is to park your directive with your primary physician's office, your children or loved ones, and anywhere else you can quickly retrieve it like your car glovebox. Some families use a fireproof safe in their home to store such important documents.

Now, you have a cell phone app to make it easier to provide these forms on demand. It is called www.MyHealthCareWishes.org . You can store an advance directive on your iPhone or Android phone for easy and quick retrieval. Though digitally transmitted, these documents have the same legal authority as signed and witnessed documents, according to Mr. Silkenat, president of the American Bar Association, who uses the app himself. Another digital storage service for healthcare and legal documents available 24/7 is www.MyDirectives.org.

AMA: Against medical advice

Hospitals ask patients to sign off on a form when they elect to leave the hospital or emergency room against medical advice. Be sure to check with your insurance insurer to see if this affects any charges for future care you receive after leaving AMA.

DNR and DNH Orders

Many patients with healthcare directives also have a Do Not Resuscitate (DNR) order and sometimes a Do Not Hospitalize (DNH) order. Ask about these forms from your doctor, treatment facility, or hospital. Keep a personal signed copy on hand for emergency room visits as well.

MEDIC ALERT NOTIFICATION

If you have a chronic disease or life threatening allergy or serious mental health condition that you want to alert any first time responder, the medic alert system is one to consider. The medic alert bracelet or necklace is inscribed with the name of your condition, medical device, allergy, or special instructions. This is especially important if you were ever in an unconscious state and unable to advocate for your personalized care. Common inscriptions can be allergy to X, asthma, pacemaker, defibrillator, medical device name, DNR, DNH, etc. The registry maintains your information for first time responders who encounter your necklace or bracelet.

MEDICAL RECORDS POLICY

We already discussed the importance of open records review to remove errors and update information on your medications or allergies. But who actually owns your medical record? I was surprised to discover that medical practices own the physical medical record with your protected health information in it. In the state of Virginia where I live, that is the law. Be sure to check with your state board of medicine. My discovery was made while investigating why our family practice destroyed the medical record of one of our adult children who had not visited the practice in a few years. I found this contrary to what I always believed – you had to be notified before a medical record could be destroyed.

Today, the medical record storage and destruction policy is also dictated by state law. In Virginia, medical provider practices can destroy a medical record after 6 years. The state medical board attorney informed me that the practice group must inform the members of any policy change or addition in writing or posted on their website. She also explained that many practice administrators are not always aware of the changes in the state law. Since they are not licensed, the state can't impose annual mandatory education requirements like they do with physicians and nurses. She helped me craft a written letter to the administrator asking for the policy to be posted on the practice website within 10 days. Failure to comply with the request would give me the duty to report them to the state for non-compliance. This was a teachable moment for me and the practice administrator and my desire to "educate not litigate" prevailed! After the policy was posted, I felt other families were better informed and hopefully, could prevent an "unknowing" destruction of their medical record!

RELEASE OF YOUR MEDICAL RECORDS

Now, that you understand how your protected health information is housed in a medical record stored by your provider, you need to grant them permission to release your protected health information to yourself or a third party such as a doctor or healthcare facility. Usually, you fill out a Medical Records Release form in the Medical Records office. Some outpatient departments also store some medical records. The form specifies the type of information you are releasing such as biopsy results, test results, doctors notes, surgical notes, and hospitalization notes and reports.

Please check with your facility whether the signature can be electronic via fax or email rather than in person. Also, ask about the price of xerox copies of the records to be sent. Sometimes, if you ask the provider or facility to send the records for you, the cost can be reduced. Expect all of this to dramatically change as electronic sharing of medical records becomes more widely used and available.

OWNERSHIP OF YOUR DNA: TISSUE AND LAB SPECIMANS

Anne Wojcicki, the CEO of 23andMe, was interviewed recently for a Wall Street Journal article. She stated that one of her goals is for people to control their own healthcare decisions. Her genetic testing company started in 2008 is presently working with the FDA to remove a temporary suspension on their delivery of personalized genetic health reports. Her company wants to get approved and return to selling this information directly to the consumer. Her personal agenda is to support more research studies on the connections between health and genetics. You own your DNA samples – whether it is your biopsy slides, your blood sample, or tumor tissue samples.

It is important to remember that you can always ask and be given a personal copy of any test result or procedure. You can also request second opinions on the pathology review of slides and accompanying report on your tissue samples. You just send the slides and request a new pathology report that you can compare with your original path report. It is always good to seek congruence of two independent set of eyes on the correct diagnosis. Your treatment plan is based on your diagnosis, so getting an accurate diagnosis is preeminent.

Knowing your genetic risks as we discussed in Chapter 4 allows you to take charge of your health and personalize it. As the information explosion reveals more about which therapies and drugs work best for different health problems associated with certain genetic variants, we will see more personalized treatment options.

Healthcare- Equalizer Consumer Bill of Rights

I have developed a set of rights that I feel every healthcare consumer should have in our healthcare system. These rights protect consumer interests and promote a consumer driven marketplace. These rights help us equalize the playing field and place responsibility on the healthcare marketplace to deliver transparent and accountable healthcare services and business practices. These rights also help consumers take a proactive approach to their health and healthcare costs.

Exercising these rights in our healthcare system assures consumers of quality and personalized care. Quality care is defined as safe, accessible, and affordable. It is also evidenced based (effective) and efficient. It is a consumer's right to expect such transparency and accountability.

Chapter 7 Challenge Goal: I challenge you to exercise one of the HCE Bill of Rights!

Healthcare-Equalizer Consumer Bill of Rights 2015

Right to be Informed about your Provider

You have the right to know the name, educational level, certification status of any healthcare provider, and the length of your appointment. You also have the right to a written copy of the business practices of the provider group including hospitalization options, travel restrictions, special billing fees, release of your medical information policies, and the medical record storage and destruction policy.

Right to be Informed about your Insurer

You have the right to receive clear, accurate, and complete information on how the deductible is determined, view up-to-date in-network provider lists, and receive a comprehensive summary of all benefits in your health plan as well as caps on the maximum costs to assume - before you choose the insurer.

Right to Price Transparency and Comparison Shopping for healthcare services

You have the right to a phone or written estimate of provider charges, expected insurance co-pays and deductible out-of-pocket costs for recommended treatment options. You also have the right to comparison shop for treatment providers and facilities, insurance plans, tests, procedures, medications, and medical devices.

Right to Safe and Quality care

You have the right and responsibility to participate in HCAHPS, a government mandated customer service survey with publicly available data results. You have the right to compare providers using publicly reported performance metrics like infection rates, mortality rates, patient satisfaction scores, and readmission rates.

Right to Personalize Your Care

You have the right to document your personal screening guidelines with your healthcare provider, develop a chronic disease treatment plan, initiate admission and discharge meetings to exchange important information like medication lists, list of allergies, and documents about your care preferences such as end-of-life directives.

Right to "Open Records" Data Transparency

You have the right to review your medical record for accuracy and make corrections. You also have the right to a written copy of your healthcare visit documentation (biometric measurements, diagnosis, contact information, and follow-up care recommendations) at the conclusion of your appointment.

Right to Financial Disclosures in your Healthcare Services

You have the right to ask your medical provider or hospital for disclosure about their financial ties to pharmaceutical companies and/or medical device manufacturers before you accept prescription drugs, treatments, tests, procedures or medical devices. You have the right to expect financial disclosure statements in any published and funded study you read.

Right to Privacy

You have the right to have your protected health information (PHI) kept private and confidential and to store your PHI in a medical record vault system of your choice. You also have the right to document any restrictions on access to sharing of your PHI as well as document any alternative method of communication you choose.

Right to Honest and Fair Billing Practices

You have the right to ask for a corrected bill and only pay the corrected bill. You have the right to a payment plan and fair billing practices. You have the right to expect that most insurance claims will be resolved within 30 days unless otherwise notified.

Right to Monitor and Report Healthcare Quality and Safety

You have the right to file complaints when your care has been unsatisfactory, unsafe, or unacceptable to you. You have the right and responsibility to report unsafe practices, unsafe practitioners, and unsafe medical products. You have the right to know actions taken by your state board that restricted, suspended, or revoked provider licenses. Your monitoring can protect your loved ones and your community.

Chapter 8 - Price: The Elusive Factor in Healthcare

Sunlight is the best disinfectant

> Louis Brandeis, Supreme Court Justice

We can overtake their power.

> "Song of Angry Men" *Les Miserables*

The lack of price transparency is a major hurdle for consumers trying to budget for expected and unexpected healthcare costs. When Steve Brill exposed the mystery charge-master system used by hospitals nationwide, he revealed the secret to their huge profits. This non-transparency gives them market control and domination and forces the consumer to accept services without knowing the prices. In order for consumers to take charge of their healthcare costs, it is imperative that we employ a different method for making health care decisions with known costs at all times. Cost always matters even when care is emergently needed.

A consumer driver marketplace will demand transparency in price as well as value based performance metrics prior to initiation of healthcare services. This chapter discusses how you can control your healthcare costs wisely. It also builds on the principle of employing independent metrics to assess safety and quality of care before choosing hospitals and other institutions for care. These consumer practices which we will discuss in more detail in Chapter 9 will give us new measures for care accountability and a new price sensitivity.

Here are some selected topics to demonstrate how we can transparently navigate the healthcare marketplace and get accountable and personalized care instead of bad and unwanted care.

PART 1: UNDERSTANDING YOUR HEALTH INSURANCE PLAN

Selecting Your Health Plan

There are a lot of factors to consider. Be sure to read everything available from the insurance company that gives you a quote. If you are employed, contact your insurance administrator in your human resources department if you have specific questions about how the plan works. Be sure you check whether you can keep your primary care provider (PCP) with a new plan. Is this doctor in your network or out of network? Also, be sure to find out what hospitals are in network and out of network in case you need hospitalization. Also, find out if there are preferred urgent care clinics that you can visit for the standard copay amount versus paying out of pocket for urgent care. Always ask the insurer how their deductible works in a particular plan.

Understanding How Your Health Plan Works

Once you enroll in a new health plan, spend time to understand how the deductible works, what copays are expected and where your up-to-date provider network list can be found. You also need to understand the cost incurred for out-of- network provider visits. You may elect to go out-of- network if you want a second opinion from a specialist outside your normal network of physicians.

If you need a colonoscopy or other screening procedure, find out whether the full cost is covered. Unfortunately, only a screening colonoscopy is usually covered completely. Once you have an established history of polyps or other high risk factors like a family history of colon cancer, your gastroenterologist's office may code your procedure as "diagnostic" not "screening." Your insurer may cover the procedure with a different level of coverage and you may be billed for a portion of the cost. Be sure to call in advance and ask your insurer and provider office what out-of-pocket costs to expect. Again, if you choose an out-of-network provider or out-of-network facility, the costs to you may be higher. If you are double insured, such as a private insurance plus Medicare, be sure to ask your doctor's office to submit any remaining amounts to the secondary insurer before billing you.

Use Your Healthcare Card Wisely

Your health insurance card usually lists a member services phone number on the front of your card. This number can be very helpful to you as you navigate the plan requirements. This number is your opportunity to make your insurance plan work for you! This is the number to call for any number of services:

Get pre-treatment copays and deductible amounts that may apply

Get expected out-of-pocket expenses for out-of-network care

Find an in-network provider from an accurate online listing available to representatives

Check the status of hospital or ER doctors who may be out-of-network even though the hospital is in-network

Find transport costs associated with a transfer of care to another facility

Some plans also have a phone number to pre-authorize ER visits and initiate behavioral health or mental health serviccs. Know how to use your health plan when travelling out of the area, as well as, out of the country.

Uninsured Care Options

Those who choose not to purchase insurance, for whatever reason, may find themselves facing extremely high prices for the care they receive. As Steve Brill's investigative team revealed, the **uninsured are billed the highest rate, the self-pay rate.** Insurance companies broker an arranged set price with hospitals and physician groups in advance.

These set prices are then built into your insurance plan. Without this brokering process, you lose out. So, if you find yourself in this predicament, I have a few suggestions.

Check with local free care clinics in your neighborhood and ask them what hospital or physician groups work with them in making referrals. When you are seen in these free clinics, they refer you to a specialist within their referral network. The price is usually less than you would pay as a self-pay patient. So, take advantage of the networks these free clinics have already arranged for needy patients. Our public health system in the US has a state network of medical and dental clinics to serve the poor and uninsured. Be sure to check your state health website to find these services in your county or state. It is important to get recommended vaccines and immunizations as well as routine dental care to keep healthy and avoid long term problems from neglected care. Prevention is always a better economic investment than waiting to treat a serious complication.

Part II: BUDGET FOR HEALTHCARE EXPENSES

The proactive approach to health also applies to the cost of healthcare services. Consumers need to be responsible for budgeting for expected healthcare costs each year. Taking charge of your budget will reduce your financial stress and maybe improve your mental health! Your monthly cost for your health plan is most likely a fixed amount. Then, you need to project how much for copays in a given year. Base this projection on your past year use of healthcare services, i.e. how many doctor or urgent care visits for you or your family. Next, find out how much a deductible you will need to cover before benefits are paid by the insurer. If you have access to a flexible spending account (FSA) for health care costs from your employer, use it.

The FSA, a tax-deferred account, is a good way to cover these costs in advance. Consider covering the maximum deductible amount with your FSA. However, today many high deductible plans may have a deductible threshold that exceeds the IRS limit of $2500. Be wise and carefully review the current IRS regulations on what these costs can cover and what expenses they don't cover. You may also be required to send in receipts from your flexible spending account administrator, so save your receipts.

Healthcare receipts

After you design your healthcare budget, keep track of all your healthcare expenses so you can forecast a better estimate for future healthcare expenses in the next year. Saving receipts also makes documentation of flexible spending costs easier and helps determine when you have reached your maximum deductible amount. Be sure to call your insurance plan and document this with them. Once this is documented, the insurer has the responsibility to pay more of your expenses that previously were applied to your deductible. In family plans with several family members or with a high expense surgery or procedure, this can happen quickly.

PART III: COMPARISON SHOP FOR PRICE AND QUALITY

As consumers become more price sensitive due to larger co-pays and higher deductible plans, this will exert a positive effect on price transparency and keeping costs down. Here are some helpful websites to compare prices of health plans, tests, procedures, and treatments:

Healthcare Bluebook

This website promotes good decisions for your health and your wallet. The website guides the consumer to the fair price for a procedure, test, or surgery in your area by zipcode. The site also offers guidance in asking your healthcare provider for the best possible price and how to use and understand your health insurance benefits. If you don't have insurance, you can download a contract to negotiate a set fair price with a local provider for a certain procedure, test, or surgery in your area. Healthcare Bluebook also offers a free pharmacy discount card and reduced fees on many standard laboratory tests.

Be sure to click on www.healthcarebluebook.com to get all this helpful information as you navigate your present and future needs for health care services.

MediBid system

This is a newcomer service for consumers seeking pre-treatment estimates across the country. If you have a high deductible health insurance plan, you may want to visit their website (www.medibid.com) to see how the program works.

This online service for consumers allows them to solicit bids from doctors and facilities. Medibid encourages its users to do their homework and research provider and facility credentials first. Chris Hobbs, its chief financial officer, believes that when patients behave like smart consumers, prices come down. The demand for this type of service is definitely growing. Many consumers with high deductibles are looking for bids before they spend their dollars on tests and procedures they need. These models encourage competition among providers. The winners usually have the best price and quality and the losers don't get much business.

Grand Rounds (grandroundshealth.com)

One of the newer healthcare startup companies is the brainchild of radiologist Lawrence "Rusty" Hoffmann. For $200, Grand Rounds, will match you with a top-ranked specialist in your area for a second opinion, schedule an office visit, supervise the transfer of your medical records and have its own physician follow-up with you. For a higher fee, usually about $7500, Grand Rounds will help you get an expert opinion from a specialist it selects. Many clients come to Grand Rounds through their employers, which often cover part of their expenses. However, Medicare and private insurers do not cover some types of second opinions.

Drug Costs

A September 2013 Consumer Report article, "Surprising Ways to Cut Your Drug Costs," had some excellent advice for healthcare consumers. Here are some of their tips:

Try an **over the counter (OTC) drug for common health problems** like heartburn, insomnia, seasonal allergies, migraine headaches, and joint pains. It is important to remember that many of these OTC drugs were once prescription only. They are usually less expensive than newer prescription drugs for the same condition.

Multi-symptom cold medications might not provide the relief you want and could cause side effects. Getting plenty of sleep and drinking lots of fluids can be very effective in helping a cold heal. Some products use antihistamines to relieve a runny nose, but increase the risk of undesirable side effects like drowsiness, dry eyes and mouth, and fluid retention.

Shop carefully and compare your insurance co-pay for generic drugs versus without the co-pay. Three month supplies of many common generic drugs can usually be bought for $10 at most major chain drugstores.

Be a smart shopper and **examine over the counter drugs on lower shelves versus the "bulls-eye" location on the top shelves with new more expensive drugs.**

Be aware of formulary changes. Every drug plan has a list of covered drugs called the formulary. Drugs not on the formulary usually have the highest out-of-pocket costs to consumers. Employers have started updating their formularies every few months in contrast to the yearly changes in the past. Sometimes, you can ask your doctor to prescribe another drug on your formulary to save money.

Your pharmacist can also be helpful in finding a different drug that is more affordable.

Call local drug stores and pharmacies and ask for the lowest price possible for the drug you plan to purchase. Sometimes you can enroll in the **pharmacy discount program** at an annual cost of $20 and save substantially on various drugs.

Use your **insurer's preferred pharmacy or mail-order service.** Usually these services have been deeply discounted by mail-order or retail pharmacy. Some insurers have struck great deals with their preferred pharmacy with deals as low as $2/month for certain generics.

Consider step therapy with a new diagnosis of a chronic condition. Newly diagnosed high blood pressure, high cholesterol, and arthritis can sometimes be treated initially with lifestyle changes – remember your RNA healthy habits– rest/sleep, nutrition and activity level. Next, your doctor may order a cheaper generic drug first to see if it is effective in controlling the condition before ordering a more expensive brand name drug.

Last, but most important**, consider taking fewer drugs**. As we have discussed in past chapters, some alternative therapies can be very effective such as acupuncture, exercise, massage, and relaxation training for back pain instead of muscle relaxants and painkillers. Taking fewer drugs also reduces your risk of side effects and possible dangerous interactions between drugs. Once a year sit down with your healthcare provider and evaluate each drug, supplement and vitamin you take and decide whether to continue.

Bartering

The ancient art of bartering prices may still be alive even in healthcare! Recent articles discuss trying the usual cash reduction of 5 or 10% as a starting point for your negotiations when paying upfront with cash! In other industries, cash sales are welcome and encouraged. So, maybe it is time to try it in healthcare! If you pay with cash instead of plastic, the provider or merchant gets the entire price.

PART IV: RESOLVE BILLING AND INSURANCE CLAIMS ERRORS

My personal and professional experience with medical bills and insurance claims is that both systems have a high and unacceptable rate of errors. So, always investigate any claim denials especially for covered services and any billing code that doesn't make sense to you. Here are some tips as you review your insurance Estimate of Benefit (EOB) reports and provider bills that contain fees or codes you didn't expect.

Medical Bill Paying Advocacy Services

Pat Palmer, the 1997 founder of Medical Billing Associates Advocates, admits that the error rate in medical billing may be as high as 80%. A smart consumer attitude is "buyer beware" to find the error on your bill before you submit payment. The hospital industry unlike the hotel industry bills separately for each item or service. Hotels quote a set price and then add fees for extra services like mini-bar purchases. Hospitals bill for each Kleenex, plastic cup, warmed blanket, etc. that you use during your visit. The expensive prices seem unwarranted and unrealistic like $150 for a warm blanket, as Steve Brill noted in his seven month investigation in 2013. You are wise to view inpatient hospitalization as well as outpatient surgical center bills line by line to review the charges carefully.

Medical Billing Associates offers the following consumer recommendations;

Examine every bill carefully looking for errors or duplication of items

Reconcile amount owed with your EOB – Explanation of Benefits report from your insurer

Keep your insurer accountable to honor their contractual obligations in your health plan. Never pay for a covered service in your plan.

Report any evidence of double billing fraud or abusive billing practices.

However, the ACA has built in **value purchasing with bundled prices for the future**. So, perhaps future hospital billing will be more straightforward and clear with one set price for the surgery, etc. Won't that be a positive change!!

Provider Representative

My own experience resolving billing and claim errors has revealed some other strategies. Each provider has a "provider representative" that works to resolve issues for consumers between the provider and your insurer. These provider reps can join your phone conversation with your provider or insurer and give helpful information. For instance, I continued to receive old bills from an insurer stating a past due balance. The provider rep was able to determine that the insurer was using an outdated address for where out-of-state claim payments were mailed. The provider representative spoke directly to the insurer and discovered the problem and solved it. My old bills stopped!!

Quality Auditor

Another resource I discovered is a quality auditor who works for your insurer. After questioning why my insurer had paid my screening mammogram and annual physical claims and then retracted the payment, my insurance representative referred me to a quality auditor. There were actually two errors! The date of the mammogram was mistakenly entered and my insurer had conducted a routine audit of my account using the wrong insurance information. This resulted in the insurer erroneously withdrawing the payment to my primary care provider. Fortunately, we were able to conduct a three-way phone call with the quality auditor and my provider to explain the error. The auditor agreed to fax a statement to my PCP office noting that my insurer was responsible for the costs not me. She informed me that providers have 72 hours to resubmit a corrected bill for payment by the insurer. My past due bill notices stopped! Now, that's service!

Old bills are another consumer nightmare in healthcare. I received an 18 month old "balance due" bill that I thought had already been paid. My first call to my insurer verified the date that a final payment had been submitted to the provider. When I called the provider back to double check the accuracy of their bill statement, I asked to speak to a supervisor. I expressed my concern that this appeared to be a case of double billing since my insurer verified payment The supervisor rechecked her files and then admitted that they must have been mistaken. **Again, check the facts with insurers first and insisting on proper and fair billing practices so we can reduce unnecessary out-of-pocket costs. Always insist on a corrected bill statement showing a zero balance by email or mail.**

Don't Forget to Document!

It is very important to keep a notebook and pen nearby when you call billing and insurance representatives. I usually document the date, time, first name of the representative, and what information they gave me or verified. Often, claims are denied for clerical or coding errors made by the provider or insurer. My insurer once told me I was their quality assurance since I found so many errors!

Coding errors are common and can occur with changes in office staff. My encounter with this problem occurred during my monthly allergy shots regimen. After a few months, I started getting billed for an additional out of pocket expense and called the billing department. A new employee had been miscoding the allergy shots and triggered the wrong benefit coverage with more out of pocket expense. I also learned that allergy shots delivered in an allergist office are billed at the higher copay amount for a specialist. You can save money receiving allergy shots from a primary care provider with a lower copay for the same service! **Lesson learned – always question anything on a bill especially a change in the usual expense for the same office visit and procedure.**

As a young clinical nurse at NIH, we attended a risk management in-service and were reminded that" it didn't happen if it isn't documented." So, written documentation is your best defense when you base a healthcare decision on information you were given by a provider or insurance representative or supervisor. Documentation of errors can also help responsible providers and insurers retrain their employees to avoid such errors in the future.

PART V: FINANCIAL TRANSPARENCY

As the healthcare transparency and accountability movement grows, consumers are becoming more aware of the financial conflicts of interest that doctors, hospitals, and medical device makers can have that influence their treatment recommendations. We need financial transparency as well as price and performance metric transparency in healthcare. Our job is to ask for the financial disclosure we need or seek it from public sources.

Financial Conflicts of Interest Information

Smart consumers need to follow the money in physician payments to determine whether there is a financial incentive for the treatment recommendation or the research study conclusions. Be sure to look at the financial disclosures at the end of clinical study results and decide whether you trust the conclusions to be impartial. Here are some websites to monitor physician payments from pharmaceuticals and medical device makers:

www.propublica.org

www.who'smydoctor.com

The Sunshine Act of the ACA

The Affordable Care Act of 2010 (ACA) has a section that required implementation of **Transparency Reports and Reporting of Physician Ownership or Investment I**

Interests. This Sunshine Act requires manufacturers of covered drugs, devices, biological products and medical supplies to report to CMS (Centers for Medicare and Medicaid Services) payments, ownership, investment interests and other transfers of value to physicians and teaching hospitals. **The intent of the law is to bring sunlight to illuminate the potential conflicts of interest with the goal of decreasing healthcare costs with such perverse incentives.**

CMS began data collection on August 1, 2013 and submitted their first report on March 31, 2014. CMS published the data on a public website in September 2014 for all consumers to read. www.cms.sunshineact.gov.

www.cms.gov/openpayments/ . **You can search by doctor name.**

Dangers of Perverse Incentives

Perverse incentives in healthcare doesn't just muddy the waters for impartial treatment recommendations, but weaves its way in business practices of price opaqueness, aggressive bill collection services, surprise facility and hidden fees, and miscoding with the most profitable code versus the correct one in fraud cases. Alert and vigilant consumers can be the first line of defense against these business practices. We need to ask lots of questions and be willing to say "no" to services we don't want and business practices that are unfair and dishonest. The more difficult issues like the pharmaceutical sales of drugs for unapproved uses to doctors for kickbacks will require legislative changes and strong enforcement to fix. Consumers, can inform providers that we value their professional integrity to disclose any and all financial strings before we receive their services.

Doctor owned healthcare businesses like imaging and surgical centers are another area of concern for financial conflicts. Many times these healthcare centers depend on surgical volume and put pressure on their doctor owners to become businessmen instead of doctors. Four recent Government Accountability Office (GAO) reports have documented a greater number of procedures by doctors who own health businesses compared to non-owner doctors. These business incentives can result in surgical overuse and sometimes recommending procedures that won't help patients.

Dr. James Rickert, an Indiana University School of Medicine faculty member, founded the Society for Patient Centered Orthopedic Society several years ago to appeal to a surgeon's conscience and encourage him/her to change their ways. Orthopedic surgeries involve serious risks for patients such as deep vein thrombosis, infections, bleeding, and nerve pain. Patients need to be informed of both the risks and benefits of a recommended surgery. Some of his fellow orthopedists have compiled a list of frequently performed procedures that are usually unnecessary, high cost, and sometimes harmful:

Vertebroplasty to repair fractured vertebra at a cost of 10K

Rotator cuff repair in elderly patients at a cost of 15K

Clavicle fracture repair or "plating" in adolescents at a cost of 13K

Anterior cruciate ligament tear repair in low risk people at a cost of 10K

Surgical removal of part of a torn meniscus at a cost of 6K

Let's reduce the influence of money in our healthcare system by getting second opinions and asking our providers to disclose their financial strings before we accept any care. It will take a long and sustained effort to create the changes in our broken American healthcare system. But together as united healthcare consumers, we can create a consumer driven marketplace that delivers safe, quality and affordable care.

Beware of Hidden Fees

It always seems ironic to me that our providers and insurers demand complete honesty and transparency about our health history as well as employment and marital status information. Yet these same providers and insurers lack transparency in their coded receipts for care, price quotes, and business practices with various fees added to our bills. Let's fight for shared transparency!

Part VI: STOP UNWANTED CARE

Only the consumer can stop unwanted care that is offered to them. You can simply refuse it. Care that does not reflect your values or budget or treatment goals is not personalized care. It is the opposite – unwanted and excessive care. You always have a right to question any drug you will be given or test that is ordered for you in a hospital or emergency room and refuse it. End of life care in hospitals is often filled with multiple tests, drugs, and procedures in an attempt to save a patient's life. Always have a care advocate – someone who will ask lots of questions and record the answers for you – when you have a care visit. The only stupid question my dad used to remind us is the "one you don't ask!!"

Healthcare Consumers can stay informed by visiting the **Choosing Wisely Campaign and Consumer Reports on Unnecessary tests and procedures websites** that were introduced in Chapter 5. It is always important to dialogue with your healthcare team to personalize your own recommended screening guidelines especially if you are high risk due to a genetic, family history, or personal risk factor for certain diseases.

For instance the **Choosing Wisely Campaign from the American Academy of Nursing** recommends **five things Nurses and Patients should question:**

Don't automatically initiate continuous electronic fetal heart rate or FHR during labor for women without risk factors; consider intermittent auscultation (IA) first

Don't let older adults lay in bed or only get up to a chair during their hospital stay

Don't use physical restraints with an older hospitalized patient

Don't wake the patient for routine care unless the patient's condition or care specifically requires it

Don't place or maintain a urinary catheter in a patient unless there is a specific indication to do so

Choosing Wisely List for American Academy of Hospice and Palliative Medicine

Don't recommend feeding tubes in patients with advanced dementia; instead offer oral assisted feeding.

Don't delay palliative care for a patient with serious illness who has physical, psychological, social or spiritual distress because they are pursuing disease directed treatment.

Don't leave an implantable cardioverter-defibrillator (ICD) activated when it is inconsistent with the patient/family goals of care.

Don't recommend more than a single fraction of palliative radiation for an uncomplicated painful bone metastasis.

Don't use topical lorazepan (Ativan), diphenhydramine (Benadryl), haloperidol (Haldol) "ABH" gel for nausea. Using these may delay or prevent the use of more effective interventions.

Chapter 8 Health Challenge Goal: I challenge you to get a pre-treatment cost quote.

Top Ten List: Smart Health Care Consumer Financial Rules for 2015

Examine each health bill carefully looking for errors to correct before you pay

Compare bills from providers after reviewing your insurer's EOB for expected payment due

Use your Provider Representative to resolve any billing errors and receive a corrected bill before rendering payment

Employ a Quality Auditor if necessary to resolve denied claims for covered services in your health plan. Be sure to get resolution before paying final bill

Ask for upfront cost estimates, in-network status, and out of pocket costs from your insurer and provider before accepting a tests, procedures, medical devices, or treatment

Manage your flexible spending account carefully. Keep receipts for each expense and be sure they comply with the latest IRS rules.

Track your deductible payments and once you have reached the maximum for yourself or the family limit, notify the insurer, and verify the expected insurer coverage for the rest of the year.

Create a health care family budget composed of health plan monthly costs and expected copay estimates and any deductibles to be met before full insurer coverage is available.

Document the date, name of representative, and action taken with each phone encounter with your provider or insurer.

Verify out of area or out of country service coverage with your plan administrator before travel

Chapter 9: Consumer Monitoring and Reporting

Eternal vigilance is the price of liberty.

Thomas Jefferson

Smart healthcare consumers must demand safe, quality care that is affordable and accessible. Such consumer vigilance assumes the willingness to report bad care, impaired providers, faulty medical devices, and unfair billing and claims review practices.

Once consumers become price sensitive and use performance metrics wisely, the providers, insurers, and medical device makers will become more transparent and accountable in their delivery of their healthcare services. Consumers are the checks and balance within the healthcare system to keep the system honest, transparent, and safe and assures better quality health outcomes.

This consumer vigilance gives the consumer powerful leverage in a provider based healthcare delivery system. Perverse incentives can make it financially profitable to increase volume instead of rewarding performance based on safety, quality, and fair pricing. Such a performance based system will allow the system to get rid of poor performers that betray the public trust by their deceptive and dishonest practices and threaten the public's health.

HEALTHCARE MONITORING FOR CONSUMERS

Medical and Pharmacy and Nursing Boards

Every state has a board of medicine, board of nursing, and board of pharmacy to protect its citizens from unlicensed providers, illegal practice activities, and impaired providers. These state boards can be contacted by consumers without initially reporting the practice or provider. It is the agency to contact to find out what the state law says about the practice or act that you are concerned about possibly reporting.

As I discussed earlier, my experience with a state board was positive. I was able to protect the identity of our family physician practice and merely inquire about what actions could be taken to resolve the medical record destruction problem we encountered. Unless consumers take action, these problems will continue. When healthcare consumers monitor the professional and safe behaviors of individual providers and their business practices, we protect our own health and the health of our communities. When you experience a problem with a practice administrator, enlist the support of your provider. Many of the senior doctors are invested partners and a non-compliance report to the State Board of Medicine or loss of a longstanding patient is not something they wish to have happen. All of these boards are available online through your state.gov website.

Reporting Unsafe Drugs, Supplements, and Faulty Medical Devices

The Food and Drug Administration (FDA) is responsible for protecting the public from unsafe drugs, supplements, and medical devices. A 2006 Institute of Medicine Report recommended the creation of a new FDA advisory committee comprised of consumers and patients to communicate with the public. This committee is tasked with assisting the public with science based information they need to use drugs, foods, supplements, and medical devices to improve their health.

In the **Recalls and Alerts** section of the FDA website, you can discover what has been recalled, withdrawn from the market, and check for posted safety alerts. There is also a section on **Medication Safety Tips** for older adults, advice on how to dispose of unused medication, and an email address to contact them at Consumerinfo@fda.hhs.gov. As you navigate the website, you will see an option to protect yourself on the consumer webpage. This link will take you to FDA's Monthly MedWatch Safety Alerts reports. Follow the link for reporting a problem, and you will find **MedWatch: the FDA Safety Information and Adverse Event Reporting Program**.

Here you can report a problem with a medical product, dietary supplement or tobacco product problem online. You can also report unlawful sales of medical products on the internet. You can download the Consumer friendly reporting **Form 3500B** in a pdf file. The FDA also encourages consumers to step forward and report voluntary adverse events that they track. This can be done so the person harmed can remain anonymous.

DailyMed is a service of the National Library of Medicine that gives current drug prescribing information. If a **drug is marked "unapproved" on this site, it means it has not been reviewed by the FDA for safety and efficacy.** They also provide **Medication Guides** which are paper handouts with specific issues for particular drugs that contain **FDA approved information to help patients avoid serious adverse reactions.**

A **2006 Institute of Medicine Report** on "The Future of Drug Safety: Promoting and Protecting the Health of the Public, **mandated that the FDA register clinical trial results to facilitate public access to drug safety information.** In 2008, the FDA shifted authority on drug safety regulatory issues to a shared partnership with the FDA Office of New Drugs (OND) with the Office of Surveillance and Epidemiology (OSE). Now, **pharmaceutical and university sponsors of Phase 2**

through 4 clinical trials are required to register in a timely manner on the National Library of Medicine website and include a summary of the efficacy and safety results of the study. So, as recommended to you in Chapter 5, the www.pubmed.gov website is an excellent search for the latest clinical trial results.

Consumer Reports in May 2012 exposed the dangerous market for faulty medical devices for consumers. They recommend consumers do their homework before the purchase of a recommended medical device. **Believe it or not, medical devices aren't tested before they hit the marketplace.** Public Citizen cited this lack of advance safety testing on trans-vaginal mesh for women with incontinence disorders when the FDA finally recalled the medical device recently. Most of these devices also lack a unique identifier like a serial number to trace them back to the consumer who owns the device once the device has been recalled. The present system relies on your doctor notifying you. What if your doctor is retired or dead?

Here are the wise recommendations that Consumer Reports suggest to protect the unsuspecting healthcare consumer:

Research the device and get the exact name of the device, brand name, model and serial number if available from your doctor/provider hospital.

Check the FDA website for consumer warnings or recalls on the device

Consider alternatives with your MD or provider

The Consumers Union, the advocacy arm of Consumer Reports (CR) agrees with the Institute of Medicine's (IOM) assessment that the current medical devices regulation doesn't protect the patient/consumer from harm. Here are their suggestions:

Insist on testing similar to drugs

End the "grandfathering clause" for new implants and life sustaining devices that don't need safety testing prior to sale

Create a unique identification system like serial numbers so consumers will be notified quickly about recalls and safety problems

Increase the regulatory fees paid by manufacturers for regulatory services

Accreditation Agencies

All health care organizations must be accredited and licensed to provide health care. These accreditation agencies also accept patient or consumer reports regarding bad care experiences particularly when patient harm has been experienced. Many healthcare offices and facilities are accredited with the **Joint Commission on Accreditation for Healthcare Organizations or JACHO.** This organization began in its gold seal approval rating system in 1951 after visiting healthcare organizations and judging them against established standards and procedures. Each organization is given a report after the visit and a rating of conditional or full approval or rejection of accreditation. When an organization receives a "conditional" accreditation, they are given time to retrain and revamp the organization before the reevaluation visit.

The quick links on their website, www.jointcommission.org/general-public brings you to the page to **Report A Complaint about a Health Care Organization.** Follow the link for the form to use and the information that you will need to register the complaint. Another link directs you to a new initiative, **Speak Up.** This campaign encourages the public to take an active role in preventing healthcare errors by becoming an informed participant in their healthcare team. These patient brochures and an info-graphic discuss important topics like anesthesia and sedation, home care, behavioral health care, and laboratory tests. The brochures describe how you can step forward and prevent errors and report them if they occur.

Here are some of the titles of their **Speak Up Brochures**

What you should know about memory problems and dementia

What you should know about adult depression

Diabetes: Five ways to be active in your care in the hospital

Information for Living Organ donors

What you should know about stroke

Five things you can do to prevent infection

Help avoid mistakes in your surgery

Help prevent errors in your care

Help prevent medical test mistakes

Know your rights

Planning your follow-up care

Reduce your risk of falling

Tips for your doctor visits

What you should know about serious illness and palliative care

Assuring lab and test results are actually your results

JACHO also lists accredited international health organizations if you are travelling abroad and provides a quality checklist of accredited and certified healthcare organizations in your area.

These are some of the areas that accreditors examine in their accreditation process for health facilities:

Infection rates and practices

Mortality statistics

Patient injury and harm statistics

As smart health care consumers, we need to fight for safe and quality care from our community healthcare organizations. Consumers have a responsibility to inform hospitals and other facilities when they have been the victims of unacceptable or dangerous care. Otherwise, how do we rid the system of the poor and dangerous performers who endanger the health of our communities?

In a consumer driven health care marketplace, consumers report errors and unsafe or poor quality care have consequences. This forces poor performing healthcare providers to accept responsibility and be accountable. This is how we can safeguard the safety, quality, accessibility, and affordability of healthcare in our communities.

Reporting Healthcare Fraud

We already recognize the huge cost of Medicare and Medicaid and other health care fraud in the US. Let's take our responsibility seriously in preventing such fraud. One obvious benefit is the revenue it will generate to fund a highly performing and efficient healthcare system! The US Office of Management and Budget states that Medicare paid more than **$47.8 billion in improper payments in 2010. This is actually 10% of the annual expenses for Medicare**.

The FDA website has several links to fraudulent sale of unsafe drugs and supplements and also informs the public about fraudulent practices in their communities and online. The Centers for Medicaid and Medicare (CMS) are working hard to track and enforce legal consequences for fraudulent care practices. They list a toll free number, 1-800-581-1790 to report healthcare fraud. The website lists the most **common types of Medicare fraud:**

Hospice care centers overbilling for patient stays and care

Rehabilitation centers systematically inflating rehab bills

Medical equipment kickback schemes for sale of bedding and wheelchairs

Nursing home overbilling of staff time and patient care

Assisted living center fraud

Medical coding changes for different procedures and diagnosis

Ambulance service fraud billing for rides not authorized by Medicare

Health insurers are also tracking fraud. You have probably noticed the instructions on how to report a fraudulent code or claim at the bottom of your Explanation of Benefits

(EOB) reports. Be sure to use this service if you suspect any fraudulent care.

If you have questions about fraudulent errors on provider bills, call the customer service department listed on the bill and report it. As you read in the last chapter, be a smart healthcare consumer and ask for a revised bill before submitting payment.

Unlawful Debt Collection Practices

Following our fiscal crisis of 2007-2008, The Dodd-Frank Wall Street Reform and Consumer Protection Act created the Consumer Financial Protection Bureau (CFPB). This bureau was created in 2011 and works in partnership with the Federal Trade Commission (FTC) to enforce fair consumer practices by financial service companies. Be sure to visit the CFPB website, www.consumerfinance.gov, which gives the consumer important information in the Fair Debt Collection Practices Act. Mr. Richard Cordray, CFPB Director, reminds consumers that debt collectors must refrain from using abusive debt collection practices and treat consumers fairly, with dignity, and prompt them to effective ways to pay their legitimate debts. In fact, 24% of all consumer complaints are due to third-party debt collectors. We all know that many healthcare organizations employ such debt collection servicers. Debt collection agencies are required to send consumers a **written notice** with the amount of debt, the name of the creditor, and a statement that they have **30 days to dispute the debt** in **writing. Unfortunately, some consumers never receive this notice**. If the consumer files a written dispute, the debt collector must stop collection efforts until it has provided the written verification of the debt. Billing departments must now include a transparent statement on how to get information on financial assistance or apply for a payment plan. Be sure to speak up if you need a payment plan and make the request in writing.

The IRS websites states that **62% of bankruptcies today are medical bankruptcies** due to unpaid medical bills. Medical billing occurs in a cycle and sometimes consumers will continue to be billed after they have paid. Be sure to call and ask for verification of payment in writing and ask the billing department to cease collection efforts. Enlist the assistance of medical billing advocates to pay your legitimate bills so this doesn't happen. Bankruptcy poses many significant restrictions on your ability to make purchases with lenders as well as negatively impact some employment opportunities and adversely affects your credit score.

Credit Agency Reporting of Medical Debt

Fortunately, we have good news about this consumer debt problem. It seems the New York states attorney office reached an agreement with three credit agencies – Transunion, Experian,and Equifax to delay reporting of medical debt before it affects a person's credit rating. This new agreement has been extended to all states and will begin implementation in 2016.

HCAHPS Program (Hospital Consumer Assessment of Healthcare Providers and Systems)

In Chapter 7, we reported on the new initiatives by CMS to solicit consumer satisfaction scores. It is vitally important to participate in this national hospital survey after your admission so we can demand safe, quality care in our communities. Let your hospital know that you care about this survey results and ask them for their latest survey results before you enter for care. Consumers want excellent health and economic value for their hard earned health dollars.

Quality Metrics to Choose Our Healthcare Facilities

A highly performing and efficient healthcare system must champion consumer choice in the marketplace and increase the transparency of publicly reported data to compare prices as well as safe and quality care outcomes among competitors. As we discussed in past chapters, we now have several options for comparison shopping for healthcare services.

For review, here is a list of some new price and performance metric websites to visit:

www.healthcarebluebook.com

www.MediBid.com

www.cms.gov/hospitalcompare

www.leapfrog.com

www.healthgrades.com

www.truvenanalytics.com

Remember no one hospital or facility is always excellent in all types of care. Seek information from other consumers and determine what values are most important to you as you make your selection. Find the provider or facility that matches your care priorities and has the expertise you need. Getting second opinions helps you meet a prospective provider and decide whether you find trust and confidence in the care they want to provide. You always want to use some independent quality and safety metrics or hard data in addition to subjective data like consumer experiences. Both are important to make informed and wise decisions.

Consumer monitoring as we learned in Chapter 8 is also about following the money in healthcare. Perverse incentives can promote unwanted and expensive care, sometimes limit consumer choice, increase out of pocket costs, and deliver poor care outcomes. Carefully consider whether financial interests are compromising the providers you interview or are recommended to you. Do your homework and check the following websites to **follow the healthcare dollars:**

www.propublica.org

www.csm.sunshineact.gov

www.whoismydoctor.com

Ultimately, each consumer is responsible for making informed healthcare decisions. Asking questions, doing your research, and expressing your desires for care preferences and personalized treatment will become the norm soon in American healthcare. Spend your healthcare dollars wisely by stopping unwanted care.

Chapter 9- Health Challenge Goal: I challenge you to participate in a HCAHPS survey after your next hospitalization and ask for your hospital's HCAHPS scores before your hospitalization.

Chapter 10: The Best is Yet to Come

Your task is not to foresee the future, but to enable it.

Antoine St Exupery, **The Little Prince**

If we have no peace, it is because we have forgotten that we belong to each other.

Mother Teresa

Will you join in our crusade?
Who will be strong and stand with me?
Beyond the barricade, is there a world you long to see?
There is a life about to start when tomorrow comes!

"Do You Hear the People Sing," *Les Miserables*

We are witnessing a new frontier in American healthcare: a trend in transparency and accountability that is most beneficial for the consumer. This trend is the healthcare-equalizer that we need to exercise our rights to receive quality, affordable, and accessible care without undue commercial influence. With every right comes a responsibility. For healthcare consumers, that responsibility is to monitor our healthcare system for safety, quality and financial disclosure. The **historic ACA law has ushered a transformation of our disease-based medical model and replaced it with a prevention based model of care system. Our fee-for-service business model and its perverse incentives on volume care is now replaced with a fee-for-value based bundled price business model**. This model incentivizes better health outcomes based on evidence for effectiveness and efficiency and patient satisfaction.

These dramatic changes will shift the allocation of resources for our personal as well as national costs for healthcare. A prevention based healthcare system rewards healthy behaviors and health promotion activities. Employers, insurers, and providers will now engage consumers on RNA topics: sleep quality and quantity, balanced diet, and regular exercise or physical activity. This new healthcare system will emphasize continual improvement with shorter timelines on release of new evidence for diagnosis and treatment of diseases and conditions. As a public health professional, this is the change in healthcare that I have strived to achieve. I believe this can lead our country to improved quality of life, increased longevity, and less disability from chronic disease. This is the good fight answer to the "root causes" of our broken healthcare system and poor health outcomes.

I hope this book has educated you about our healthcare system and motivated you to take charge of your health and healthcare decisions. Our health status is closely tied to our quality of life. It makes sense that our health care services reflect our quality of life goals and values. We are entering an age of the consumer which can transform our healthcare system to a consumer driven marketplace. We have many technological advances to allow us to measure our biometrics by ourselves and choose when, where, and how much to pay when we need healthcare services. In fact, the locus of control in the healthcare marketplace is no longer in the hands of providers, but rather in our own hands! This is a powerful responsibility that we must accept.

Consumers need to make smart decisions about healthcare by understanding our body, our healthcare rights, and be proactive about our health risks. This new mindset also embraces treatment for the "root causes" of our symptoms and chronic diseases to achieve better control and possibly a cure. Consumers in the driver's seat for their healthcare decisions can minimize "controllable" health risks and promote screening tests and procedures to monitor our "uncontrollable" health risks.

Personalized healthcare is on the horizon as well. This healthcare is not just about using our DNA to diagnose our health risks, but also includes DNA sampling of our healthcare threats for the most effective treatment. In my opinion, **personalized healthcare is care that reflects our personal risks as well as our cultural and religious values, care preferences, and our own definition of quality of life.** Vocal consumers who are educated and informed will drive our healthcare system to better health outcomes, less cost, and greater efficiency. It is imperative that we join the good fight and create a highly performing American healthcare system.

My Healthcare-Equalizer Consumer Bill of Rights is my effort to support the important role of consumers in the healthcare marketplace. As consumers take charge of their own health and healthcare decisions, they will also say no to unwanted care, excessive care, expensive care and bad care. Healthcare consumers must know what quality of life they want and insist on the healthcare providers respecting their values and care preferences. More consumers will have written documents to frame palliative care desires and end-of-life wishes. Smart consumers will insist on an honest assessment of the benefits and risks of treatment options before making their decisions.

Let's vow to make Health our number 1 national priority. This will require a public health mandate that looks to streamline our system of care and get rid of inefficiencies, excesses, and ineffective ways of delivering care. My public health mandate for better healthcare outcomes in the US involves three steps:

Step One: Healthy Communities

Step Two: Legislation Initiatives

Step Three: Proactive Healthcare Consumers

Step One: Healthy Communities

Healthy People 2020 – Take Charge and Create a Healthy Community

The 1979 Surgeon General's Report on health promotion and disease prevention began this movement. The Healthy People 1990 was the first report to focus on national health objectives to achieve health promotion and disease prevention goals outlined in the Surgeon General's Report. Today these science-based 10-year national objectives aim to improve the health of all Americans. It encourages collaboration across communities and regions of the country as well as empowers individuals to make informed health decisions. Most importantly, it measures the impact of various prevention activities.

The Healthy People 2020 framework emphasizes the dynamic influence of personal, environmental, organizational, and policy determinants of health and health behaviors. The report advocates the need for schools and communities to foster preventive health measures and create healthy physical environments. The 2020 objectives also stress the role of **health information technology and health communication to measure and support its successful implementation**.

The launch of Healthy People 2010 followed the September 11, 2001 attack, anthrax incidents, several natural disasters, and global influenza concerns. This report recognized the urgency of preparedness as a public health issue. **The 2020 Report adopted the term "all hazards" as its all-encompassing approach.**

The Healthy People 2020 Model (issued in 2010) continues a focus on population group disparities in health outcomes due to race/ethnicity, socioeconomic status, gender, age, disability status, sexual orientation and geographic location. Its overarching goals include:

Attain high quality, longer lives free of preventable disease, disability, injury, and premature death

Achieve health equity, eliminate disparities, and improve the health of all groups

Create social and physical environments that promote good health for all

Promote quality of life, healthy development, and healthy behaviors across all life stages

Step Two: Public Health Legislation Works

Good health is always about the interdependence between our internal and external environments. Healthy air and water as well as healthy food and habits improve the health of a state and nation. Prevention is economically and socially responsible.

The 2010 Institute of Medicine Report on "Avoidable Healthcare Costs" advocates sharing big data scientific study conclusions quickly to change evidenced based guidelines as soon as possible so better health outcomes are continuously improved. The newly established **Patient Care Outcomes Research Institute (PCORI)** has a mandate to accomplish this under the ACA. Just as our diagnosis and treatment guidelines are updated and improved, our public health laws must also follow suit to protect the health of our citizens.

Air Pollution vs. Heart Attack and Stroke Incidence

Two 2012 studies in the Journal of the American Medical Association and the Archives of Internal Medicine examined the effect of short term pollution exposure (1-7 days) on the incidence of heart attack and stroke in people with predisposing respiratory and heart diseases. It appears there is no safe level of pollution. The **exposure risk increases in time and intensity. Heart attacks and stroke rates rise after high-pollution days, especially for those with predisposing conditions. The heart attack risk rose almost 5% with high carbon monoxide levels and almost 3% with higher levels of air particles for up to seven days.**

The most troublesome particulate tiny droplets are PM2-58. These particles emanate from power plants, factories, trucks and cars. Fine particulate matter (dust, soot, smoke and liquid droplets) are particularly dangerous to human health because they can lodge deep in the lungs causing respiratory diseases and cancer according to the EPA. A **2013 Lancet,** a British Medical Journal, **study found the incidence of heart failure also rises when air pollution is higher. So, a reduction of PM2.5 can reduce hospitalizations due to heart failure in the US with cost savings of approximately $330,000,000 per year.** Lastly, a study of air pollution in Northern China by the Proceedings of National Academy of Sciences suggested life expectancy could be lowered by as much as 5.5 years.

Monitoring air quality makes health sense for healthy communities. Electric powered vehicles may yield much cleaner air in communities in the future. Many local weather reports now routinely track various allergens for their viewers and readers. Here is an app from the Environmental Protection Agency (EPA) that works on both Apple and Android cellphones. It gives the user pollutant and ozone levels for morethan400 cities across the country:

www.AIRNOW.org

Smoking Ban

A 2010 NCI (National Cancer Institute) study examined the effect of smoking bans in casinos on the number of ambulance calls. A smoke-free law was implemented in July 2006 and was extended to include casinos in Colorado in 2008. A study in the journal, *Circulation,* noted a **20% decreased incidence of cardiac and pulmonary events, commonly follow the enactment of smoke-free laws in local areas.** Another novel study found a **31% increase in ambulance calls following the opening of 24 -hour casinos**. This study noted that only 19 states and Puerto Rico require state-related casinos to be smoke free. Their recommendation was to **apply smoke-free laws to all casinos to lower ambulance calls as well as healthcare cost reductions to states.**

Trans Fat Labeling Changes

Researchers at the CDC discovered the effect of **trans-fat blood levels** following the FDA labeling regulations in 2003. The National Health and Nutrition Examination Survey found significant measurable health changes following this labeling change. **Between 2000 and 2008, the blood level of trans-fat declined by 58%.** During this time period, several parts of the country including New York passed state or local laws limiting the amount of trans-fats used in restaurant food and cooking. The makers of some processed foods voluntarily replaced these cheap trans-fats like palm oil and coconut oil with less harmful oils like canola, olive or corn. **By 2008, 98% of restaurants had stopped using trans-fats in oils, shortenings and spreads compared to 50% before the regulation.**

The Need for Health Insurance Reform legislation

While doing research for this book and after listening to patients, I am convinced that mandatory health insurance reform is necessary to control our healthcare costs and improve the efficiency and effectiveness of our healthcare system. In Chapter 1, we learned that the US health insurance industry has a 110% greater administrative costs than any other country. This is due to our complex and fragmented insurance system. We need much more transparency in health plan descriptions prior to purchase, mandatory updating of network provider lists monthly, and more accountability for insurers to guide their insured members with decisions across care transitions. This will most likely necessitate 24/7 coverage like the automobile and housing insurance industries already provide. Consumers need assistance navigating their health plans when accidents, serious illness, and hospitalizations occur. They need transparent discussions about coverage, deductibles, and expected out- of- pocket costs associated with various decisions they make.

Dr Makary makes the case in his book, **Unaccountable,** that the healthcare industry isn't accountable to the public like other industries. A personal experience with our house insurance company made me think the same thing. Bad things don't just happen to our car and house, they happen to our bodies, too and deserve the same level of quality and service accountability.

During Hurricane Isabel in 2011, our neighbor's 110 foot tall poplar tree crashed through our brick sunroom and adjoining deck. We were awakened at 4am by a loud bang and rushed downstairs to find rain gushing through our beautiful breakfast room soaking the hardwood floors in the adjacent kitchen. A heap of debris surrounded a 3 foot diameter poplar trunk had broken a hole in the hardwood floor and exposed our basement gym to rainwater and debris.

Our frantic 4am phone call to our homeowners insurance company was answered quickly by a calm and extremely helpful customer service insurance representative. She notified us about our policy coverage, our $1000 deductible, and instructed us to get the tree trunk removed and tarp the sunroom as soon as possible to limit further water damage. She also reminded us that the sooner the tree was removed, the sooner the structural damage could be assessed. After multiple meetings with the claims adjuster, structural engineer, and various cost estimators to repair the damage, we negotiated a fair and honest insurance claim settlement 60 days later. Car, home, and health insured members need information and service 24/7. Every healthcare decision has both a financial as well as health outcome.

Step Three: Proactive Healthcare Consumers

There is a better way to deliver healthcare in America and it begins with educated and informed healthcare consumers. A consumer driven health care system is at the heart of a prevention based care delivery system. The consumer is the hub of the system and demands safe, quality, transparent, affordable, and accountable care.

We have our work cut out for us! It will require a host of new **advocacy skills for healthcare consumers:**

Adopt smart health daily habits

Comparison shop for price, quality and safety

Keep a healthcare family budget

Support our quality of life values in all our healthcare decisions including advanced directives

Monitor the system and report bad care and outcomes

Take Charge of Our Health

Health is a long term investment with a foundation of healthy, daily habits. The health triangle is built on healthy nutrition, an active lifestyle, and quality sleep and relaxation. These healthy behaviors will decrease stress in our lives, improve our biometric measurements, and prevent or reduce the impact of many chronic diseases. Our bodies, by design, must move daily, eat nutritious food and our mind needs periods of relaxation, rest, and a sense of community.

Here are my **Healthcare-Equalizer Consumer responsibilities** in this new frontier in American healthcare:

Action One: Seek out the root cause of chronic symptoms and treat it.

Action Two: Practice self-care with biometric monitoring and self-manage chronic disease to stay as healthy as possible and avoid complications and hospitalizations. Develop your own RNA and Chronic Disease Action Plan as well as personalized screening guidelines with your provider.

Action Three: Budget for expected healthcare costs and seek financial transparency about each and every healthcare decision you make. Stay in network for most services to control your costs.

Action Four: Use public (independent) health metrics on healthcare quality, safety, and price to make wise, informed decisions about where to go for safe, quality care and how much to pay.

Action Five: Support preventive health efforts in your community, workplace, and schools.

Action Six: Take charge of communication with health team at each care transition point - emergency room, hospital, rehab facility, assisted living, dementia facility, nursing home, or hospice. Initiate admission and discharge meetings to communicate your clear care expectations and preferences.

Action Seven: Report bad care and insist on actions to prevent such bad care in the future from providers. Participate in patient surveys, ask for HCAHPS results, and give feedback on what you expect.

Action Eight: Insist on price and data transparency from your insurer before you decide on recommended tests or treatments. Fight denied claims that involve usually covered services.

Action Nine: Keep a "buyer- beware" attitude and look for errors in billing and claims filed. Most likely you will find one that needs to be resolved prior to your bill payment.

Action Ten: Insist on care that you want and need and reflects your definition of quality of life.

Mr. Schiller, the Yale behavioral economist who won the 2013 Nobel Economics prize, remarked that human behavior matters and irrational markets need vigilant consumers. Maybe our present irrational healthcare market with its "perverse incentives" will meet its match when consumers insist on transparency and accountability with each and every healthcare decision they make.

Exercise your Healthcare-Equalizer Consumer Bill of Rights. You can review them at the end of this book.

Part Four: The Best is Yet to Come – Our Future Healthcare System

Let's imagine what our future healthcare system might look like! It will reward healthy lifestyles with reduced cost of insurance like safe drivers. It will diagnose chronic diseases at an early stage where treatment is most effective and the cost is minimal. It will respect consumer quality of life values and care preferences. It will build healthy communities who keep providers and insurers accountable to consumers with honest business practices, affordable safe and quality care without fraud, unwanted, and bad care.

This health care transformation can deliver a much more effective public good – safe, quality health care services at an affordable price by partnering with data and informatics technology. www.datapalooza.com is a website analyzing the health data revolution that has just started. We are witnessing the transition from an opaque, closed and proprietary system for health care data that is rapidly becoming more transparent and open. Data will be shared across many organizations in health with the national health care IT movement generating electronic medical records. This data transparency of publicly reported data on healthcare price, quality, safety, and as well as patient data and clinical trial and funded study results will unleash a ripe environment for consumers to take charge of their health and healthcare decisions and create a consumer driven marketplace. These forces can transform our present healthcare system with its perverse incentives and emphasis on disease to a prevention based healthcare system focused on health and wellness as well as highly performing and efficient.

Just imagine,

A future where you can compare providers by quality and safety metrics in your community

A future where you can ask or get financial disclosure or seek public information on pharmaceutical or medical device strings attached to your provider or healthcare facility.

A future where you can choose your healthcare plans online instead of just through an employer

A future where researchers share data so we can understand what works and what doesn't work more quickly and translate that into evidenced based practices for care

A future where technology allows patients to monitor and self-manage their biometrics and communicate with their providers electronically from home and prevent complications

A future where your screening tests, treatment choices, and end-of-life decisions are all personalized by you based on your DNA, personal values, and personal preferences

In summary, **Thomas Edison was right – there is a better way and we have found it – reform the American healthcare system with transparency and accountability! Together, we can create a consumer driven marketplace and highly performing healthcare**

system. Let's aim to be the global leader in healthcare outcomes!

Please join this new frontier in American healthcare. Become an informed and educated healthcare consumer. Please visit my website at https://healthcare-equalizer.com

Chapter 10 Health Challenge Goal: I challenge you to increase your level of physical activity this month, record how you feel and act, and measure one biometric for changes!

Healthcare-Equalizer Consumer Bill of Rights 2015

Right to be Informed about your Provider

You have the right to know the name, educational level, and certification status of your healthcare provider and the length of your appointment. You also have the right to a written copy of the business practices of the provider group including hospitalization options, travel restrictions, special billing fees, release of your medical information policies, and their medical record storage and destruction policy.

Right to be Informed about your Insurer

You have the right to receive clear, accurate, and complete information on how the deductible is determined, view up-to-date in-network provider lists, a list of covered and uncovered services, and receive a comprehensive summary of all benefits including caps on the maximum costs to assume before you choose the insurer.

Right to Price Transparency and Comparison Shopping for Healthcare Services

You have the right to a written estimate of provider charges, expected insurance co-pay and deductible out-of-pocket costs for recommended treatment option. You also have the right to comparison shop for healthcare providers, insurance plans, tests, procedures, medications, and medical devices.

Right to Safe and Quality care

You have the right to participate in HCAAPS, a nationally mandated customer service survey with publicly available data results. You have the right to compare providers using publicly reported performance metrics like infection rates, mortality rates, patient satisfaction scores, and readmission rates.

Right to Personalize Your Care

You have the right to document your personal screening guidelines with your healthcare provider, develop a chronic disease treatment plan, initiate admission and discharge meetings to exchange important information like medication lists, list of allergies, and documents about your care preferences and end-of-life directives.

Right to "Open Records" Data Transparency

You have the right to review your medical record for accuracy and make corrections. You also have the right to a written copy of your healthcare visit documentation (biometric measurements, diagnosis, contact information, and follow-up care recommendations) at the conclusion of your appointment.

Right to Financial Disclosures in Your Healthcare Services

You have the right to ask your medical provider or hospital for disclosure about their financial ties to pharmaceutical companies and/or medical device manufacturers before you accept prescription drugs, treatments, tests, procedures or medical devices. You have the right to expect financial disclosure statements in any published and funded study you read.

Right to Privacy

You have the right to have your protected health information (PHI) kept private and confidential and to store your PHI in a medical record vault system of your choice. You also have the right to document any restrictions on access to sharing of your PHI as well as document any alternative method of communication you choose.

Right to Honest and Fair Billing Practices

You have the right to ask for a corrected bill and pay after you receive a corrected bill. You have the right to a payment plan and fair billing practices. You have the right to expect that most insurance claims will be resolved within 30 days unless otherwise notified.

Right to Monitor and Report Healthcare Quality and Safety

You have the right to file complaints when your care has been unsatisfactory, unsafe, or unacceptable to you. You have the right to report unsafe practices, unsafe practitioners, and unsafe medical products. You have the right to know actions taken by state boards to restrict, suspend, or revoke provider licenses. Your monitoring can protect your loved ones and your community.

About the Author

Rita A. Rooney is a professional nurse with 40 years of experience in a variety of healthcare settings. She earned her Bachelor of Science degree in Nursing from the University of Delaware with honors in 1975. Rita received the Madeline McDowell Award for high competence in professional nursing at graduation and was inducted into the Sigma Theta Tau International Nursing Honor Society.

In 1980, she earned a Master of Public Health degree from Johns Hopkins University with an emphasis on Healthcare Administration and Health Education. Rita earned the Blue Pencil Award from the National Association of Government Communicators for the development of the Breast Cancer Patient Education Series in 1982. She was honored with an Exemplary Service Award from Georgetown University Hospital Healthcare Referral Department in 1998.

Rita and husband, Frank, live in Arlington and have three adult children. Rita enjoys travel, gardening, geneology, and mysteries!